**Workbook
to
Accompany**

Introduction to Health Science Technology

BLAHH____

**Workbook
to
Accompany**

Introduction to Health Science Technology

Louise Simmers, M.Ed., R.N.

THOMSON

DELMAR LEARNING

Australia   Canada   Mexico   Singapore   Spain   United   Kingdom   United States

Workbook to Accompany Introduction to Health Science Technology

Executive Director:
William Brottmiller

Executive Editor:
Cathy L. Esperti

Acquisitions Editor:
Sherry Gomoll

Senior Developmental Editor:
Marah Bellegarde

Executive Marketing Manager:
Dawn F. Gerrain

Channel Manager:
Jennifer McAvey

Editorial Assistant:
Jennifer Conklin

Art/Design Coordinator:
Connie Lundberg-Watkins

Project Editor:
Bryan Viggiani

Production Editor:
Anne Sherman

Library of Congress Catalog No. 2002041715
ISBN 1-4018-1129-9

International Divisions List

Asia (Including India):
Thomson Learning
60 Albert Street, #15-01
Albert Complex
Singapore 189969
Tel: 65 336-6411
Fax: 65 336-7411

Australia/New Zealand:
Nelson
102 Dodds Street
South Melbourne
Victoria 3205
Australia
Tel 61 (0)3 9685-4111
Fax 61 (0)3 9685-4199

Latin America:
Thomson Learning
Seneca 53
Colonia Polanco
11560 Mexico, D.F. Mexico
Tel: (525) 281-2906
Fax: (525) 281-2656

Canada:
Nelson
1120 Birchmount Road
Toronto, Ontario
Canada M1K 5G4
Tel (416) 752-9100
Fax (416) 752-8102

UK/Europe/Middle East/Africa:
Thomson Learning
Berkshire House
1680-173 High Holborn
London WC 1V 7AA
United Kingdom
Tel 44 (0)20 497-1422
Fax 44 (0)20 497-1426

Spain (includes Portugal):
Paraninfo
Calle Magallanes 25
28015 Madrid
España
Tel 34 (0)91 446-3350
Fax 34 (0)91 445-6218

Notice to the Reader

Publisher does not warrant or guarantee any of the products described herein or perform any independent analysis in connection with any of the product information contained herein. Publisher does not assume, and expressly disclaims, any obligation to obtain and include information other than that provided to it by the manufacturer.

The reader is expressly warned to consider and adopt all safety precautions that might be indicated by the activities described herein and to avoid all potential hazards. By following the instructions contained herein, the reader willingly assumes all risks in connection with such instructions.

The publisher makes no representation or warranties of any kind, including but not limited to, the warranties of fitness for particular purpose or merchantability, nor are any such representations implied with respect to the material set forth herein, and the publisher takes no responsibility with respect to such material. The publisher shall not be liable for any special, consequential, or exemplary damages resulting, in whole or part, from the readers' use of, or reliance upon, this material.

CONTENTS

CHAPTER 14 FIRST AID

CHAPTER 15 PREPARING FOR THE WORLD OF WORK

PART 5: WORKING IN HEALTH CARE

CHAPTER 16 COMPUTERS IN HEALTH CARE

TO THE STUDENT

Two different types of worksheets are provided in this workbook: assignment sheets and evaluation sheets. These sheets are designed to correlate with specific information and procedures discussed in the textbook, *Introduction to Health Science Technology*.

The assignment sheets are designed to allow you to review the main facts/information about a procedure. After you read the information about a specific procedure in the textbook, try to answer the questions on the corresponding assignment sheet. Refer to the information in the text to obtain the correct answers to the questions or statements. Then check the information to be sure your answers are correct. Let your instructor grade the completed assignment sheet. Note any points that are not correct. Be sure you understand these points before you perform the procedure. This will provide you with the basic knowledge or facts necessary before a procedure is done.

The evaluation sheets are designed to set criteria or standards that should be observed while a specific procedure is being performed. They follow the steps of the procedure as listed on the procedure sections in the textbook. As you practice each procedure, use the specific evaluation sheet to judge your performance. When you feel you have mastered a particular procedure, sign the evaluation sheet and give it to your instructor. The instructor will use this sheet to grade you on your performance.

The format of the evaluation sheet is designed to provide for both practice and the final evaluation of the procedure. The appearance of the evaluation sheet and the meaning of each of the abbreviations and parts is as follows:

HST Evaluation Sheet

Name _____   Date _____

Evaluated by _____

DIRECTIONS:

Name of Procedure	Points Possible	Peer Check Yes No	Final Check* Yes No	Points Earned**	Comments

PROFICIENT

Name: Sign your name in this area.

Date: The date you are given your final evaluation can be placed in this area.

Evaluated by: The person who is evaluating you (usually the instructor) on your final check of this procedure will sign his/her name in this area.

Directions: Basic directions for using the sheet are provided in this area.

Name of Procedure: The specific name of the procedure will be noted in this area.

Points Possible: A number will appear in this column—beside each step of the procedure. The number represents the points you will receive if you do this step of the procedure correctly.

Peer Check: These columns are used for practice when your peer (another student) watches as you perform the procedure. If you complete the step correctly, the peer (student) should check the "Yes" column. If you omit a step, or do not complete it correctly, the peer (student) should check the "No" column. After you complete the procedure, you can use this checklist as an indication of steps completed correctly and those needing additional practice.

Final Check: These columns will be used by the person (usually the instructor) doing your final check or evaluation on the procedure. Two columns are provided, one labeled "Yes" and one labeled "No." If you perform a step of the procedure correctly, the evaluator will place a check in the "Yes" column. If you do not perform a step of the procedure, or perform a step incorrectly, the evaluator will place a check in the "No" column.

Points Earned: In this column the evaluator will give you the correct number of points (as stated in the "Points Possible" column) for each step of the procedure on which you received a check in the "Yes" column. You will not receive the points for a particular step if you received a check in the "No" column. The number of points earned can then be totaled. A grade can be assigned by a scale determined by your instructor.

Comments: This column is for comments regarding your performance of the procedure. Any check in the "No" column should be explained by a brief explanation opposite the step in which the error occurred. In addition, positive comments on your performance of the procedure should be noted in this area.

As you can see, the evaluation sheet provides you with an opportunity to actually practice your performance test on a particular procedure before you have to take the final performance evaluation. By utilizing this sheet, you will achieve higher standards of performance and learn to master all steps of each procedure.

The sheets in this book follow the same order of procedures/skills found in the textbook. Each information section in the textbook refers you to a specific assignment sheet in the workbook. Each procedure section in the textbook refers you to a specific evaluation sheet in the workbook. By following the directions in the textbook and the directions on each of the sheets in this workbook, you can master the procedures/skills and become competent health worker.

Matrix of Skills Used in Health Occupations
&
Correlation to National Health Care Skill Standards

Matrix of Skills Used in Health Occupations

SKILLS	CLINICAL LABORATORY SERVICES	DENTISTRY	DIETETICS AND NUTRITION	EDUCATION	HEALTH INFORMATION AND COMMUNICATION	HEALTH SERVICES ADMINISTRATION	MEDICINE	MENTAL, PHYSICAL, SOCIAL SPECIALTIES	NURSING	PHARMACY	PODIATRY	SCIENCE AND ENGINEERING	TECHNICAL INSTRUMENTATION	VETERINARY MEDICINE	VISION CARE
Chapter 1: Health Care Systems															
History of health care	X	X	X	X	X	X	X	X	X	X	X	X	X	X	X
Private health care facilities	X	X	X	X	X	X	X	X	X	X	X	X	X	X	X
Government agencies	X	X	X	X	X	X	X	X	X	X	X	X	X	X	X
Voluntary or nonprofit agencies	X	X	X	X	X	X	X	X	X	X	X	X	X	X	X
Health insurance plans	X	X	X	X	X	X	X	X	X	X	X	X	X	X	X
Organizational structure	X	X	X	X	X	X	X	X	X	X	X	X	X	X	X
Trends in health care	X	X	X	X	X	X	X	X	X	X	X	X	X	X	X
Chapter 2: Careers in Health Care															
Introduction to Health Careers	X	X	X	X	X	X	X	X	X	X	X	X	X	X	X
Dental careers		X		X	X										
Diagnostic services	X	X	X	X	X	X	X	X	X	X	X	X	X	X	X
Emergency medical services	X	X	X	X	X	X	X	X	X	X	X	X	X	X	X
Health information and communication services	X	X	X	X	X	X	X	X	X	X	X	X	X	X	X
Hospital/health care facility services	X		X	X	X	X	X	X	X	X	X				
Medical careers				X			X	X	X		X				X
Mental and social services				X	X	X	X	X	X						
Mortuary careers				X	X	X	X	X	X						
Nursing careers				X	X	X	X	X	X		X				
Nutrition and dietary services		X	X	X	X	X	X	X	X						
Therapeutic services	X	X	X	X	X	X	X	X	X	X	X	X	X	X	X
Veterinary careers				X	X									X	
Vision services				X	X	X	X	X	X	X			X		X
Chapter 3: Personal Qualities of a Health Care Worker															
Personal appearance	X	X	X	X	X	X	X	X	X	X	X	X	X	X	X
Personal characteristics	X	X	X	X	X	X	X	X	X	X	X	X	X	X	X
Teamwork	X	X	X	X	X	X	X	X	X	X	X	X	X	X	X
Professional leadership	X	X	X	X	X	X	X	X	X	X	X	X	X	X	X
Stress	X	X	X	X	X	X	X	X	X	X	X	X	X	X	X
Time management	X	X	X	X	X	X	X	X	X	X	X	X	X	X	X
Chapter 4: Legal and Ethical Responsibilities															
Legal responsibilities	X	X	X	X	X	X	X	X	X	X	X	X	X	X	X
Ethics	X	X	X	X	X	X	X	X	X	X	X	X	X	X	X
Patient's rights	X	X	X	X	X	X	X	X	X	X	X	X	X	X	X
Advance directives for health care	X	X	X	X	X	X	X	X	X	X	X	X	X	X	X
Professional standards	X	X	X	X	X	X	X	X	X	X	X	X	X	X	X

Matrix of Skills Used in Health Occupations

SKILLS	CLINICAL LABORATORY SERVICES	DENTISTRY	DIETETICS AND NUTRITION	EDUCATION	HEALTH INFORMATION AND COMMUNICATION	HEALTH SERVICES ADMINISTRATION	MEDICINE	MENTAL, PHYSICAL, SOCIAL SPECIALTIES	NURSING	PHARMACY	PODIATRY	SCIENCE AND ENGINEERING	TECHNICAL INSTRUMENTATION	VETERINARY MEDICINE	VISION CARE
Chapter 5: Medical Terminology															
Using medical abbreviations	X	X	X	X	X	X	X	X	X	X	X	X	X	X	X
Interpreting word parts	X	X	X	X	X	X	X	X	X	X	X	X	X	X	X
Chapter 6: Anatomy and Physiology															
Basic structure of the human body	X	X	X	X	X	X	X	X	X	X	X	X	X	X	X
Body planes, directions, and cavities	X	X	X	X	X	X	X	X	X	X	X	X	X	X	X
Integumentary system	X	X	X	X	X	X	X	X	X	X	X	X	X	X	X
Skeletal system	X	X	X	X	X	X	X	X	X	X	X	X	X	X	X
Muscular system	X	X	X	X	X	X	X	X	X	X	X	X	X	X	X
Nervous system	X	X	X	X	X	X	X	X	X	X	X	X	X	X	X
Special senses	X	X	X	X	X	X	X	X	X	X	X	X	X	X	X
Circulatory system	X	X	X	X	X	X	X	X	X	X	X	X	X	X	X
Lymphatic system	X	X	X	X	X	X	X	X	X	X	X	X	X	X	X
Respiratory system	X	X	X	X	X	X	X	X	X	X	X	X	X	X	X
Digestive system	X	X	X	X	X	X	X	X	X	X	X	X	X	X	X
Urinary system	X	X	X	X	X	X	X	X	X	X	X	X	X	X	X
Endocrine system	X	X	X	X	X	X	X	X	X	X	X	X	X	X	X
Reproductive system	X	X	X	X	X	X	X	X	X	X	X	X	X	X	X
Chapter 7: Human Growth and Development															
Life stages		X	X	X	X		X	X	X	X					X
Death and dying			X	X	X	X	X	X	X			X	X	X	
Human needs	X	X	X	X	X	X	X	X	X	X	X	X	X	X	X
Effective communication	X	X	X	X	X	X	X	X	X	X	X	X	X	X	X
Chapter 8: Nutrition and Diets															
Fundamentals of nutrition	X	X	X	X	X	X	X	X	X	X	X	X	X	X	X
Essential nutrients	X	X	X	X	X	X	X	X	X	X	X	X	X	X	X
Utilization of nutrients	X	X	X	X	X	X	X	X	X	X	X	X	X	X	X
Maintenance of good nutrition	X	X	X	X	X	X	X	X	X	X	X	X	X	X	X
Therapeutic diets		X	X	X			X	X	X					X	
Chapter 9: Cultural Diversity															
Culture, ethnicity, and race	X	X	X	X	X	X	X	X	X	X	X	X	X	X	X
Bias, prejudice, and stereotyping	X	X	X	X	X	X	X	X	X	X	X	X	X	X	X
Understanding cultural diversity	X	X	X	X	X	X	X	X	X	X	X	X	X	X	X
Respecting cultural diversity	X	X	X	X	X	X	X	X	X	X	X	X	X	X	X

Matrix of Skills Used in Health Occupations

SKILLS	CLINICAL LABORATORY SERVICES	DENTISTRY	DIETETICS AND NUTRITION	EDUCATION	HEALTH INFORMATION AND COMMUNICATION	HEALTH SERVICES ADMINISTRATION	MEDICINE	MENTAL, PHYSICAL, SOCIAL SPECIALTIES	NURSING	PHARMACY	PODIATRY	SCIENCE AND ENGINEERING	TECHNICAL INSTRUMENTATION	VETERINARY MEDICINE	VISION CARE
Chapter 10: Geriatric Care															
Myths on aging	X	X	X	X	X	X	X	X	X	X	X		X	X	X
Physical changes of aging	X	X	X	X	X	X	X	X	X	X	X		X	X	X
Psychosocial changes of aging	X	X	X	X	X	X	X	X	X	X	X		X	X	X
Confusion and disorientation in the elderly	X	X	X	X	X	X	X	X	X	X	X		X	X	X
Meeting the needs of the elderly	X	X	X	X	X	X	X	X	X	X	X		X	X	X
Chapter 11: Promotion of Safety															
Using body mechanics	X	X	X	X	X	X	X	X	X	X	X	X	X	X	X
Preventing accidents and injuries	X	X	X	X	X	X	X	X	X	X	X	X	X	X	X
Observing fire safety	X	X	X	X	X	X	X	X	X	X	X	X	X	X	X
Chapter 12: Infection Control															
Understanding the principles of infection control	X	X	X	X	X	X	X	X	X	X	X	X	X	X	X
Washing hands	X	X	X	X	X	X	X	X	X	X	X	X	X	X	X
Observing standard precautions	X	X	X	X	X	X	X	X	X	X	X	X	X	X	X
Sterilizing with an autoclave	X	X	X	X		X	X	X	X	X	X	X	X	X	X
Using chemicals for disinfection	X	X	X	X		X	X	X	X	X	X	X	X	X	X
Cleaning with an ultrasonic unit	X	X	X	X		X	X	X	X	X	X	X	X	X	X
Using sterile techniques	X	X	X	X		X	X	X	X	X	X	X	X	X	X
Maintaining transmission-based isolation	X	X	X	X		X	X	X	X	X	X	X	X	X	X
Chapter 13: Vital Signs															
Measuring and recording vital signs	X	X		X			X	X	X	X	X	X	X	X	X
Measuring and recording temperature	X	X		X			X	X	X	X	X	X	X	X	X
Measuring and recording pulse	X	X		X			X	X	X	X	X	X	X	X	X
Measuring and recording respirations	X	X		X			X	X	X	X	X	X	X	X	X
Graphing temperature, pulse, and respiration (TPR)	X	X		X			X	X	X	X	X	X	X	X	X
Measuring and recording apical pulse	X	X		X			X	X	X	X	X	X	X	X	X
Measuring and recording blood pressure	X	X		X			X	X	X	X	X	X	X	X	X

Matrix of Skills Used in Health Occupations

SKILLS	CLINICAL LABORATORY SERVICES	DENTISTRY	DIETETICS AND NUTRITION	EDUCATION	HEALTH INFORMATION AND COMMUNICATION	HEALTH SERVICES ADMINISTRATION	MEDICINE	MENTAL, PHYSICAL, SOCIAL SPECIALTIES	NURSING	PHARMACY	PODIATRY	SCIENCE AND ENGINEERING	TECHNICAL INSTRUMENTATION	VETERINARY MEDICINE	VISION CARE
Chapter 14: First Aid															
Providing first aid	X	X	X	X	X	X	X	X	X	X	X	X	X	X	X
Performing cardiopulmonary resuscitation (CPR)	X	X	X	X	X	X	X	X	X	X	X	X	X	X	X
Providing first aid for bleeding and wounds	X	X	X	X	X	X	X	X	X	X	X	X	X	X	X
Providing first aid for shock	X	X	X	X	X	X	X	X	X	X	X	X	X	X	X
Providing first aid for poisoning	X	X	X	X	X	X	X	X	X	X	X	X	X	X	X
Providing first aid for burns	X	X	X	X	X	X	X	X	X	X	X	X	X	X	X
Providing first aid for heat exposure	X	X	X	X	X	X	X	X	X	X	X	X	X	X	X
Providing first aid for cold exposure	X	X	X	X	X	X	X	X	X	X	X	X	X	X	X
Providing first aid for bone and joint injuries	X	X	X	X	X	X	X	X	X	X	X	X	X	X	X
Providing first aid for specific injuries	X	X	X	X	X	X	X	X	X	X	X	X	X	X	X
Providing first aid for sudden illness	X	X	X	X	X	X	X	X	X	X	X	X	X	X	X
Applying dressings and bandages	X	X	X	X	X	X	X	X	X	X	X	X	X	X	X
Chapter 15: Preparing for the World of Work															
Developing job-keeping skills	X	X	X	X	X	X	X	X	X	X	X	X	X	X	X
Writing a letter of application and preparing a resumé	X	X	X	X	X	X	X	X	X	X	X	X	X	X	X
Completing job application forms	X	X	X	X	X	X	X	X	X	X	X	X	X	X	X
Participating in a job interview	X	X	X	X	X	X	X	X	X	X	X	X	X	X	X
Determining net income	X	X	X	X	X	X	X	X	X	X	X	X	X	X	X
Calculating a budget	X	X	X	X	X	X	X	X	X	X	X	X	X	X	X
Chapter 16: Computers in Health Care															
Introduction to computers	X	X	X	X	X	X	X	X	X	X	X	X	X	X	X
What is a computer system?	X	X	X	X	X	X	X	X	X	X	X	X	X	X	X
Computer applications	X	X	X	X	X	X	X	X	X	X	X	X	X	X	X
Using the Internet	X	X	X	X	X	X	X	X	X	X	X	X	X	X	X
Chapter 17: Medical Math															
Math anxiety	X	X	X	X	X	X	X	X	X	X	X	X	X	X	X
Basic calculations	X	X	X	X	X	X	X	X	X	X	X	X	X	X	X
Estimating	X	X	X	X	X	X	X	X	X	X	X	X	X	X	X
Roman numerals	X	X	X	X	X	X	X	X	X	X	X	X	X	X	X
Angles	X	X	X	X	X	X	X	X	X	X	X	X	X	X	X
Systems of Measurement	X	X	X	X	X	X	X	X	X	X	X	X	X	X	X
Temperature conversion	X	X	X	X	X	X	X	X	X	X	X	X	X	X	X
Military time	X	X	X	X	X	X	X	X	X	X	X	X	X	X	X

Correlation to National Health Care Standards

CHAPTER	Health Care Core Standard								Therapeutic/ Diagnostic Core					Therapeutic Cluster			
	Academic Foundation	Communication	Systems	Employability Skills	Legal Responsibilities	Ethics	Safety Practices	Teamwork	Health Maintenance Practices	Client Interaction	Intrateam Communication	Monitoring Client Status	Client Movement	Data Collection	Treatment Planning	Implementing Procedures	Client Status Evaluation
Chapter 1	X	X	X	X	X		X	X	X		X						
Chapter 2	X		X	X	X			X			X			X			
Chapter 3	X	X	X	X	X	X	X	X	X	X	X						
Chapter 4		X	X	X	X	X				X	X	X		X	X	X	
Chapter 5	X	X															
Chapter 6	X								X		X	X					
Chapter 7	X	X		X	X	X		X		X	X	X		X	X		X
Chapter 8	X								X	X				X	X		X
Chapter 9	X	X		X	X	X		X	X	X	X	X	X	X	X	X	X
Chapter 10	X	X			X	X	X	X	X	X	X	X	X	X	X		X
Chapter 11					X		X				X	X	X	X	X	X	X
Chapter 12	X				X	X	X		X		X			X		X	X
Chapter 13	X				X		X		X	X	X	X		X		X	X
Chapter 14				X	X	X				X	X	X	X	X	X	X	X
Chapter 15	X	X		X	X	X		X	X								
Chapter 16	X	X		X	X						X			X			X
Chapter 17	X			X										X	X	X	X

Correlation to National Health Care Standards

CHAPTER	Diagnostic Cluster					Information Services Cluster					Environmental Services Cluster			
	Planning	Preparation	Procedure	Evaluation	Reporting	Analysis	Abstracting and Coding	Information Systems	Documentation	Operations	Environmental Operations	Aseptic Procedures	Resource Management	Aesthetics
Chapter 1						X							X	
Chapter 2	X									X	X			
Chapter 3												X		
Chapter 4	X				X	X		X	X		X	X		
Chapter 5					X		X		X					
Chapter 6												X		
Chapter 7								X	X		X		X	
Chapter 8												X		X
Chapter 9	X	X	X	X	X	X		X	X				X	
Chapter 10		X			X							X		X
Chapter 11	X	X	X	X	X						X		X	X
Chapter 12			X	X							X	X	X	
Chapter 13	X	X	X	X	X		X		X		X			
Chapter 14	X	X	X	X	X									
Chapter 15													X	
Chapter 16					X	X		X	X	X				
Chapter 17			X			X	X	X	X	X			X	

CHAPTER 1 HEALTH CARE SYSTEMS

ASSIGNMENT SHEET

Grade ___11___ Name _Brittany Annis_

INTRODUCTION: An awareness of the many different kinds of health care systems is important for any health care worker. This assignment will help you review the main facts on health care systems.

INSTRUCTIONS: Read the information on Health Care Systems. Then follow the instructions by each section to complete this assignment.

A. Completion or Short Answer: In the space provided, print the word(s) that best completes the statement or answers the question.

1. Unscramble the following words to identify some health care facilities.

   a. RAALOTBYRO _laboratory_
   b. TLEHHA NNCIAMTNAEE _health maintenance_
   c. OLGN ETMR AREC _long term care_
   d. UNLTISIDAR ETHLAH _industrial health_
   e. MNCEGEREY AECR _emergency care_
   f. LNTEMA LHTEHA _mental health_
   g. LNCCII _clinic_
   h. EAIINRIABHTLTO _rehabilitation_
   i. POTSAHIL _hospital_

2. Place the name of the type of health care facility by the brief description of the facility.

   a. _long term care facilities_ provide assistance and care for mainly elderly patients
   b. _emergency care service_ provide special care for accidents or sudden illness
   c. _Mental health_ deal with mental disorders and disease
   d. _industrial health care centers_ health centers located in large companies or industries
   e. _dental offices_ offices owned by one or more dentists
   f. _laboratories_ perform special diagnostic tests
   g. _home health care_ provide care in a patient's home
   h. _Clinics_ provide physical, occupational, and other therapies

3. Hospitals are classified into four types depending on the sources of income received. List the four (4) main types.

   1) private/proprietary
   2) religious
   3) nonprofit/voluntary
   4) government

4. List three (3) services offered by medical offices.

— Pediatrics — Cardiology — Obstetrics

5. Identify at least three (3) different types of clinics.

— Surgical clinics — urgent/emergency care clinics
— rehabilitation clinics

6. List three (3) examples of services that can be provided by home health care agencies.

— nursing care — personal care, — therapy

7. What is the purpose or main goal for the care provided by rehabilitation facilities?

To provide care to patients with physical/mental disabilities obtain maximum self-care/function.

8. Identify three (3) services offered by school health services.

— emergency care — perform tests
— promote health education

9. An international agency sponsored by the United Nations is the *World Health Organization*.
A national agency that deals with health problems in America is the *US dep. of health & service*. Another national organization that is involved in the research of disease is the *Nat. inst. of health*.
A federal agency that establishes and enforces standards that protect workers from job-related injuries and illnesses is the *Occup. Safety & health ad*. The federal agency that researches the quality of health care delivery and identifies the standards of treatment that should be provided is the *Agency for health care policy & research*

10. List four (4) services that can be offered by state and local health departments.

— immunization for disease control — inspections for enviro. health & services — communicable disease control — collection of statistics & records

11. Nonprofit or voluntary agencies provide many services.

   a. How do these agencies receive their funding?

   — donations   — fundraisers
   — membership fees   — federal/state grants

   b. List two (2) services provided by these facilities.

   — purchasing medical equipment & supplies
   — providing treatment centers

12. Define the following terms related to insurance plans.

   a. premium: *a payment (monthly) to insurance)*
   b. deductible: *amounts that must be paid by the patients for the medical services before the policy begins to pay*
   c. 75/25% co-insurance: *requires specific percentages of the expenses are shared by the patient & insurance company*
   d. co-payment: *specific amount of money a patient pays for a particular serv*
   e. HMOs: *type of health insurance plan*
   f. PPOs: *type of health insurance plan*
   Preferred Provider Organization

Name __Brittany Annis__

13. a. What is one advantage to HMOs?

The fee stays the same regardless of the amount of health care used.

b. What is one disadvantage to HMOs?

The insured is required to use only HMO-affiliated health care providers.

14. Why has the concept of managed care developed? What is the principle behind managed care?

Developed in response to rising health care costs. The principal is that all health care provided to a patient must have purpose.

15. Identify the individuals who are usually covered under the following plans.

Medicare: almost all individuals over 65+ anyone with a disability

Medicaid: individuals with low income, children who qualify, + physically disabled or blind individuals

State Children's Health Insurance Program: uninsured children of working families who don't make enough

Workers' Compensation: workers injured on the job

16. What is the purpose for an organizational structure in a health care facility?

Encompasses a line of authority or chain of command.

17. What is holistic health care?

Care that promotes physical, emotional, social, intellectual, + spiritual well-being by treating the whole body, mind, + spirit.

18. The Omnibus Budget Reconciliation Act (OBRA) of 1987 established standards for geriatric assistants in long-term care facilities. List four (4) requirements that all geriatric assistants must meet as a result of OBRA.

- Complete a mandatory, state-approved test + pass a written examination
- continuing of education, periodic evaluation of performance
- compliments with patients/residents rights
- forces states to establish guidelines

19. Describe what is meant by the following trends in health care. Include a brief explanation of why it is important to be aware of these trends.

a. cost containment: trying to control the rising cost of health care + achieving the maximum benifit for every dollar spen

b. diagnostic related groups (DRGs): *One way Congress is trying to control costs for government insurence plans such as Medicare & Medicaide*

c. energy conservation: *monitering the use of energy to control costs & conserve resources*

d. home health care: *usually less expensive to provide this type of care*

e. geriatric care: *allows longer life spans, care for the elderly*

f. telemedicine: *decreases the need for trips to medical facilities*

g. wellness: *people are more aware to mainteen good health which saves money optimal state of health*

h. alternative and complementary methods of health care: *becoming more common alt - find methods instead of accepted treatment comp - in addition to recomended treatment*

20. Do you think a national health care plan should be established to provide coverage for all individuals? Why or why not?

Yes, our health is essential to life and everyone needs to be cared for.

Name Brittany Annis

B. Matching: Place the letter of the person in Column B in the space provided by the person's contribution to the history of health care in Column A.

Column A

C ~~X~~ 1. Isolated radium in 1910

Q 2. Established the patterns of heredity

N 3. Developed a vaccine for smallpox in 1796

L 4. Described the circulation of blood to and from the heart

V 5. Began public health and sanitation systems

U 6. Discovered X-rays in 1895

M 7. The father of medicine

I 8. Discovered penicillin in 1928

D 9. Artist who used dissection to draw the human body

E ~~B~~ 10. Emphasis was placed on saving the soul and study of medicine
was prohibited

A 11. Founded the American Red Cross in 1881

G 12. Earliest people known to maintain accurate health records

S 13. Began pasteurizing milk to kill bacteria

B 14. Used acupuncture to relieve pain and congestion

O 15. Developed the culture plate method to identify pathogens

R 16. Founder of modern nursing

P 17. Began using disinfectants and antiseptics during surgery

H 18. Created the first mercury thermometer

W 19. Developed the polio vaccine in 1952

T 20. An Arab physician who began the use of animal gut
for suture material

Column B

A. Clara Barton
B. Chinese
C. Marie Curie
D. Leonardo da Vinci
E. Dark Ages
F. Dorthea Dix
G. Egyptians
H. Gabriel Fahrenheit
I. Sir Alexander Fleming
J. Benjamin Franklin
K. Sigmund Freud
L. William Harvey
M. Hippocrates
N. Edward Jenner
O. Robert Koch
P. Joseph Lister
Q. Gregory Mendel
R. Florence Nightengale
S. Louis Pasteur
T. Rhazes
U. William Roentgen
V. Romans
W. Jonas Salk

20 - True / False
15 - Multiple Choice
10 - Matching
  - explain terms related to insurance
  - know types of insurance
  - know different types of health care agencies
  - different people (nurses, romans, egyptians...)

ASSIGNMENT SHEET

Grade _____   Name _____

INTRODUCTION: An individual who wants to work in health care has a wide variety of career choices. This assignment will help you review some of the different careers.

INSTRUCTIONS: Read the information on Careers in Health Care. Then follow the instructions by each section to complete this assignment.

A. **Health Career Search:** All the careers listed are hidden in the following word search puzzle. Locate and circle the careers.

admitting officer	home health care	pedodontics
animal technician	internist	perfusionist
athletic trainer	licensed practical nurse	pharmacist
biomedical equipment	medical laboratory	physical therapist
central supply	medicine	physician
chiropractic	music therapist	podiatric
dental hygienist	neurologist	psychologist
dentist	nurse	radiologic technologist
dialysis technician	occupational therapist	recreational therapist
dietitian	optician	respiratory therapy
doctor	optometrist	social worker
electrocardiograph	osteopathy	surgeon
electroencephalographic	orthodontics	surgical technician
emergency medical	paramedic	urologist
endodontics	pathologist	veterinarian
geriatric aide	pediatrician	ward clerk
gynecologist		

```
O R T H O D O N T I C S Z X E W P T V B P H Y S I C A L T H E R A P I S T X M N E C I D
C X V E T E R I N A R I A N O P C M I D W Q T Y P X B N N A I C I N H C E T L A M I N A
C E W I O N G H T S I G O L O N H C E T C I G O L O I D A R X B N M N I U T Y E M C T V
U M K I J T V E P B I U N J X U T Y O P H Y E P I U O P T O M E T R I S T X V M E K E L
P C V I E I T R O J K L I M U R O L O G I S T T X E M K U L I E R H W E S E S Q D X R L
A A S E T S I E D V B N T U E S M O P I E T H I R O E V U I S E D P A R A M E D I C N X
T L I E K T E R I L K E R N O E G R U S Y U R C E I D Z Q C W E A A T R G E U O C H I O
I T L M I D I C A I N E A R O T C O D T H E R I P H I X E E O R T R H E P R I K I I S L
O B O A T H L E T I C T R A I N E R E M U W T A I N C P I N C H I G R S O G P R N R T A
N P A T H E R O R G Y N P E D O D O N T I C S N P E A D O S D O N O T P I E C S E O D E
A N T I N A I T I T E I D S T N U R T H E A L T A I L Y U E R E S I P I R N A P T P R Y
L R E C G Y N E C O L O G I S T R E A A W A R D C L E R K D X T I D O R N C A E L R A I
T D P H Y S I C I A N E R N E U R O L O G I S T X Y Q R A P D I O R L A O Y G D M A I S
H N S S E U R S E X O S T E O P A T H Y O S T I O P U A T R H Y X A R T O M P I U C M N
E X Y Z W S C E N T R A L S U P P L Y S A N I T A T I J K A H O M C R O E E T A S T L S
R E C B N R T S I C A M R A H P Y O G G R O S T I E P O U C I E T O B R N D M T I I W E
A T H H E L P M E E D I A C I R T A I R E G R I G H M T O T N T O R R Y U I P R C C B O
P H O M E H E A L T H C A R E T I E E S C H O H L R E J U I T O E T M T N C C I T O I P
I X L Y O U S U R G I C A L T E C H N I C I A N F O N I U C N C S C X H P A M C H W Q R
S P O R E C E P T R E C I F F O G N I T T I M D A X T I O A Y Z D E T E C L G I E R U N
T O G E T H I E W A R D I A L Y S I S T E C H N I C I A N L M O M L R R I O P A R U R O
B N I Z Y M E D I C A L L A B O R A T O R Y T E A C H U R N V O W E X A E L M N A S E T
C X S O C I A L W O R K E R R I T W Q Y C V T S I N O I S U F R E P X P L O V I P K E N
F E T H E R B I R T S I P A R E H T L A N O I T A E R C E R E A G L O Y R E T C I H I C
A B X E N D O D O N T I C S H Y G I E N P A T H O L O G I S T V E T E R A M I X S M A L
E L E C T R O C I H P A R G O L A H P E C N E O R T C E L E X E N C A R D G R A T H I C
```

B. Matching: Place the letter of the abbreviation in Column B in the space provided by the career it represents in Column A.

Column A		Column B	
____	1. Occupational Therapist	A.	AMT
____	2. Certified Medical Laboratory Technologist	B.	CBET
____	3. Nurse Midwife	C.	CLT
____	4. Doctor of Dental Medicine	D.	CMA
____	5. Emergency Medical Technician	E.	CMT
____	6. Doctor of Osteopathy	F.	CNM
____	7. Certified Biomedical Equipment Technician	G.	CRNP
____	8. Registered Nurse	H.	DC
____	9. Optometrist	I.	DMD
____	10. Registered Dietitian	J.	DDS
____	11. Doctor of Dental Surgery	K.	DO
____	12. American Medical Transcriptionist	L.	DPM
____	13. Doctor of Podiatric Medicine	M.	DVM or VMD
____	14. Certified Medical Assistant	N.	ECG or EKG
____	15. Electrocardiograph Technician	O.	EEG
____	16. Physical Therapist	P.	EMT
____	17. Doctor of Chiropractic	Q.	LPN or LVN
____	18. Licensed Practical/Vocational Nurse	R.	MD
____	19. Doctor of Medicine	S.	OD
____	20. Nurse Practitioner	T.	OT
____	21. Certified Laboratory Technician	U.	PT
____	22. Veterinarian	V.	RD
____	23. Electroencelphalographic Technician	W.	RN
____	24. Respiratory Therapist	X.	RT

C. Completion or Short Answer: In the space provided, print the word(s) that best complete the statement or answer the question.

1. Briefly describe the educational requirements for the following degrees.

Associate's:

Bachelor's:

Master's:

2. Identify the following methods used to ensure the skill and competency of health care workers:

    a. A professional association or government agency regulating a particular health career issues a statement that a person has fulfilled the requirements of education and performance and meets the standards and qualifications established:

    b. A government agency authorizes an individual to work in a given occupation after the individual has completed an approved education program and passed a state board test:

    c. A regulatory body in a health care area administers examinations and maintains a list of qualified personnel:

3. What is the difference between a technician and a technologist?

4. Who are multicompetent or multiskilled workers?

    Why do smaller facilities and rural areas hire these workers?

5. Define *entrepreneur.*

    List three (3) characteristics of a person who is an entrepreneur.

6. The following statements describe medical or dental specialities. Print the correct name of the specialty or specialist in the space provided.

    a. _____ alignment or straightening of the teeth

    b. _____ diseases and disorders of the eye

    c. _____ diseases and disorders of the mind

    d. _____ surgery on the teeth, mouth, and jaw

    e. _____ disorders of the brain and nervous system

    f. _____ diseases of the female reproductive system

    g. _____ diseases of the kidney, bladder, or urinary system

    h. _____ illness or injury in all age groups

    i. _____ treatment and prevention of diseases of the gums

    j. _____ diagnosis and treatment of tumors

7. The following statements describe health careers. Print the correct name of the career in the space provided.

a. _____ works under supervision of a dentist to remove stains and deposits from the teeth, expose and develop X-rays

b. _____ operates machine to record electrical activity in brain

c. _____ work with X-rays, radiation, nuclear medicine, ultrasound

d. _____ provide basic care for medical emergencies, illness, injury

e. _____ organize and code patient records, gather statistical data

f. _____ manage the operation of a health care facility

g. _____ nurse assistant who works with elderly individuals

h. _____ dispense medications on written orders from others who are authorized to prescribe medications

i. _____ use recreational and leisure activities as form of treatment

j. _____ examine eyes for vision problems and defects, not an MD

k. _____ prepare a body for interment

8. Review the different health careers and find at least three careers that interest you. List the three careers and include a brief description of the duties and educational requirements of each. Also include a brief statement about why you might like to work in each career.

9. Choose one of the careers listed previously and write to an organization that will provide additional information about the career. Let your instructor check your letter before you mail it. Organizations and addresses are provided after each career cluster in the textbook. If you have access to the Internet, contact the organization by using the Internet address provided or by doing an Internet search. This will allow you to read or print a hard copy of information on the career.

... for optimum health

... ability to deal w/ stress

store: helps prevent ... have + puts less stress on muscles

... am working towards ... attitude we're being ... say + do ... position

CHAPTER 3 PERSONAL QUALITIES OF A HEALTH CARE WORKER

ASSIGNMENT SHEET

Grade _____ Name _____

INTRODUCTION: Certain personal characteristics, attitudes, and rules of appearance apply to all health care workers even though they may be employed in many different careers. This assignment will help you review these basic requirements.

INSTRUCTIONS: Read the information on Personal Qualities of a Health Care Worker. Then follow the instructions by each section and complete this assignment.

A. Crossword: Use the Key Terms for personal characteristics of a health care worker to complete the crossword puzzle.

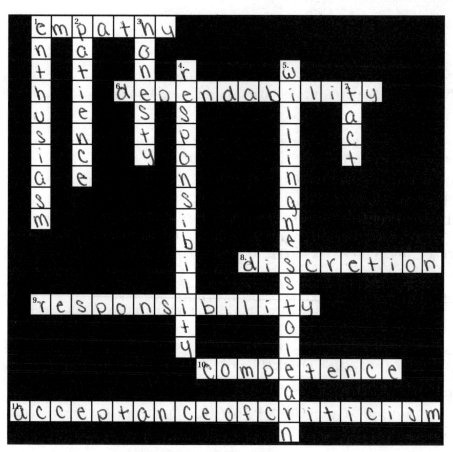

4 down - self motivation

ACROSS

1. Identify with and understand another's feelings
6. Accept responsibility because others rely on you
8. Use good judgment in what you say and do
9. Willing to be held accountable for your actions
10. Qualified and capable of performing a task
11. Accept opinions of others and learn from them

DOWN

1. Display a positive attitude and enjoy work
2. Tolerant and understanding
3. Show truthfulness and integrity
4. Ability to begin or follow through with a task
5. Adapt to changes and learn new things
7. Say or do the kindest or most fitting thing

B. Characteristic Profile: Write a characteristic profile of yourself as a health care worker that describes at least eight (8) of the personal characteristics without using the actual words. A sentence describing empathy is shown as an example.

As a health worker, I must have a sincere interest in people, and I must be able to identify with and understand another person's feelings, situation, and motives.

- I must be tolerant, understanding, + able to control my temper.
- I must show the skill + ability to encourage others to work together + do their best.
- I must be truthful and willing to admit my mistakes.
- I must have a desired goal/purpose to which I am working towards.
- I must enjoy my work and show a positive attitude.
- I must always use good judgement in what I say + do.
- I must accept the responsibility required in my position
- I must be qualified and capable of performing a task.

C. Completion and Short Answer: In the space provided, print the answer to the question or complete the statement.

1. List five (5) factors that contribute to good health and briefly describe why each factor is beneficial.

    i) Diet: provides the body w/ materials needed for optimum health

    2) Rest: provides energy + the ability to deal w/ stress

    3) Exercise: maintains circulation + provides muscle tone

    4) Good Posture: helps prevent fatigue + puts less stress on muscles

    5) Avoid use of Tobacco, Alcohol, + Drugs: helps prevent damage to the body systems

2. Identify three (3) basic requirements for the appearance of uniforms.

    1) neat

    2) well fitting

    3) clean

    4) wrinkle free

3. How do you determine which type and color of uniform to wear in your place of employment?
   - some agencies require white uniforms, some allow pastels
   - some agencies use colors to identify different groups of workers

4. List three (3) basic rules to observe in regard to shoes worn in a health career.
   1) fit well & provide good support
   2) avoid tennis shoes/sandels unless they are uniform
   3) avoid wearing high heels

5. List three (3) ways to control body odor.
   1) daily bath/shower
   2) use of deoderant
   3) good oral hygeine
   4) clean undergarments

6. List three (3) reasons why the nails must be kept short and clean.
   1) can injure patients if they are long
   2) transmit germs
   3) can tear/puncture gloves

7. What can be used to keep the hands from becoming chapped and dry because of frequent handwashing?
   - hand cream/lotion

8. Why is it important to keep long hair pinned back and off the collar when a job requires close patient contact?
   - prevents hair from touching patient/resident
   - prevents hair from falling on a tray/equipment
   - prevents hair from blocking neccessary vision during procedures

9. What jewelry can be worn with a uniform?
   - watch
   - wedding ring
   - small, pierced earrings

   Why should excessive jewelry be avoided?
   - interfere w/patient care
   - detracts from professional appearance

10. What is the purpose of makeup?
    - create a natural apperance
    - add to the attractiveness of a person

11. Define *teamwork*.

Many professionals with different levels of education, ideas, backgrounds, and intrests, working together for the benifit of the patient.

12. List five (5) ways to develop good interpersonal relationships.
- maintain a positive attitude & learn to laugh at yourself
- be friendly & cooperate with others
- assist others when you see that they need help
- listen carefully when another person is sharing ideas or beliefs

13. Briefly describe the characteristics of each of the following types of leaders:

a. democratic: encourages the participation of all individuals in decisions that have to be made / problems that have to be solved

b. laissez-faire: believes in non-interference in the affairs of others

c. autocratic: maintains total rule, makes all decisions, and has difficulty delegating/sharing duties

14. Define *stress*.

The body's reaction to any stimulus that requires a person to adjust to a changing enviroment

15. Identify the four-step plan that should be followed when a stressor causes a physical reaction in the body.
1) Stop: immediately stop what you are doing to break out of the stress response
2) Breathe: relieves physical tention you are feeling
3) Reflect: think about the problem at hand & the cause of the stress
4) Choose: determine how you want to deal with the stress

16. Identify a situation that always leads to stress in your life. Briefly describe how you can adapt to or deal with the situation to decrease or eliminate stress.
- Homework
- don't procrastinate
- set aside time to do it & get it done

17. Differentiate between short-term and long-term goals.
- Short: good grades
- long: becoming a nurse

18. List the seven (7) steps of an effective time management plan.
1) Analyze & prioritize
2) Identify habits & preferences
3) Schedule tasks
4) Make a daily "to do" list
5) Plan your work
6) Avoid distractions
7) Take credit for a job well done

CHAPTER 4 LEGAL AND ETHICAL RESPONSIBILITIES

ASSIGNMENT SHEET

Grade _____ Name _____

INTRODUCTION: All health care workers must understand the legal and ethical responsibilities of their particular health career. This assignment will help you review the basic facts on legal and ethical responsibilities.

INSTRUCTIONS: Read the information on Legal and Ethical Responsibilities. In the space provided, print the word(s) that best completes the statement or answers the question.

1. Use the Key Terms to fill in the blanks.

   a. _Contract_ (agreement between two or more parties)

   b. _tort_ (wrongful acts that do not involve contracts)

   c. _slander_ (spoken defamation)

   d. _defamation_ (a false statement)

   e. _libel_ (written defamation)

   f. _confidentiality_ (without legal capacity) *legal disability*

   g. _legal_ (authorized or based on law)

   h. _agent_ (person working under principal's direction)

   i. _ethics_ (principles morally right or wrong)

   j. _false imprisonment_ (restricting an individual's freedom)

   k. _malpractice_ (bad practice)

   l. _assault_ (threat or attempt to injure)

   m. _negligence_ (failure to give expected care)

   n. _patients rights_ (factors of care patients can expect)

2. Create a situation that provides an example that could lead to legal action for each of the following torts.

   a. malpractice: _leaving a sponge in a person_

   b. negligence: _not turning someone on bedrest_

c. assault and battery:
  • assault - threatining to physically harm a patient
  • battery - touching someone w/o their consent

d. invasion of privacy:
  exposing a patient w/o their consent

e. false imprisonment:
  keeping a patient in the hospital w/o their consent

f. abuse:
  hitting a patient

g. defamation:
  Telling people a patient has a drug problem when they don't.

3. How are slander and libel the same? How are they different?
  • Same - they are both defamation
  • different - one is spoken, the other is written.

4. What are the three (3) parts of a contract?
  1) offer: individual entering a relationship w/ a health care provider offers to be a patient
  2) acceptance: health care provider gives appt. or examines/treats patient
  3) consideration: payment is made by the patient

5. What is the difference between an implied and an expressed contract?
  • implied - obligations that are understood w/o verbally expressed terms
  • expressed - stated in distinct/clear language, either orally or written

6. List three (3) examples of individuals who have legal disabilities.
  1) minors
  2) mentally incompetent individuals
  3) individuals under the influence of drugs

7. What legal mandate must be followed when a contract is explained to a non-English-speaking individual?
  A translator must be used.

8. Why is it important for a health care worker to be aware of his/her role as an agent? Who is responsible for the actions of the agent?

- To protect the interests of their employers.
- the principal is responsible

9. What are privileged communications?

Comprise all information given to health care personnel by a patient, and by law this information must be kept confidential and shared only with other members of the patients health care team.

What is required before privileged communications can be told to anyone else?

Written consent of the patient.

10. List three (3) examples of information that is exempt by law and not considered to be privileged communications.

- births + deaths
- injuries caused by violence (abuse, assault, battery, stabings)
- drug abuses
- STD's

11. Who has ownership of health care records?

The health care provider

What rights do patients have in regard to their health care records?

They may maintain a copy

12. What should you do if you make an error while recording information on health care records?

Cross it out with a single line and the insert, initial, and date the correct information.

13. List three (3) ways health care facilities create safeguards to maintain computer confidentiality.

- limiting personnel who have access to the records
- using codes
- requiring passwords

14. What are ethics?

A set of principals relating to what is morally right/wrong.

15. What should you do in the following situations to maintain your legal/ethical responsibilities?

a. A patient dying of cancer tells you he has saved a supply of sleeping pills and intends to commit suicide.

Put the saving of life and the promotion of health above all else.
—Report it immediately

b. You work in a nursing home and see a coworker shove a patient into a chair and then slap the patient in the face.

Inform a higher authority.

c. You work as a dental assistant and a patient asks you, "Will the doctor be able to save this tooth or will it have to be pulled?"

Think before you speak and carefully consider everything you say.
—refer the question to the dentist

d. A patient has just been admitted to an assisted care facility. As you are helping the patient undress and get ready for bed, you notice numerous bruises and scratches on both arms.

Report possible abuse.

16. The factors of care that patients can expect to receive are frequently called __rights__. These state in part that a patient has the right to __recieve__ and __refuse__ care, receive __information__ necessary to give his or her __informed__ consent, refuse __treatment__ to the extent permitted by law, __confidential__ treatment of all records, reasonable __response__ to request for services, __examine__ the bill and receive a/an __explanation__ of all charges, refuse to __participate__ in any research project, and expect reasonable __continuity__ of care.

17. What is the name of the act that guarantees certain rights to residents in long-term care facilities?

~~Residents Bills of Rights~~
Omnius Budget Recgonation Act (OBRA)

18. What is the purpose for each of the following advance directives for health care?

a. Living will:

Allow individuals to state what measures should/shouldn't be taken to prolong life when their conditions are terminal.

b. Durable Power of Attorney (POA):

Allows an individual to appoint another individual to make decisions for them if they become unable to.

19. What is the purpose of the Patient Self-Determination Act (PSDA)?

Mandates that all health care facilities recieving any type of federal aid must comply with certain requirements.

20. Describe two (2) ways you can identify a patient.

- Check the name band
- State the patients name clearly

21. What should you do in the following situations to maintain professional standards?

a. The doctor you work for asks you to give a patient an allergy shot, but you are not qualified to give injections.

Perform only the procedures for which you have been trained and are legally permitted to do.

b. An elderly patient, who is frequently confused and disoriented, refuses to let you take his temperature.

~~Obtain a legal gaurdian consent.~~
Try to convince them its the best thing but don't force it.

c. You work in a medical laboratory. A patient's wife asks you if her husband's blood test was positive for an infectious disease.

Think before you speak and carefully consider everything you say. Have her talk to her husband.

22. What is a *DNR* order? What does it mean?

Do not recessitate.

Mandates that all health care facilities receiving any type of federal aid must comply with certain requirements.

CHAPTER 5:1 USING MEDICAL ABBREVIATIONS

ASSIGNMENT SHEET

Grade _____ Name _____

INTRODUCTION: Shortened forms of words (often just letters) are called abbreviations. You are probably familiar with some such as AM, which means morning, and PM, which means afternoon or evening. The world of medicine has many of its own abbreviations. At times they are used by themselves. At other times, several abbreviations are used together to give orders or directions.

As a health worker, many directions will be given to you in abbreviated form. You will be expected to know their meaning. The following assignment will assist you in starting to see how these abbreviations are used, and how you must translate them to understand them.

INSTRUCTIONS: Review the information on standard medical abbreviations. Try to recall the meanings of the following terms before using them as references to complete the exercises.

A. Print the meanings of the following abbreviations.

1. D/C _____
2. OR _____
3. prn _____
4. ac _____
5. stat _____
6. RN _____
7. wt _____
8. Cl _____
9. Rx _____
10. AP _____
11. T _____
12. NPO _____
13. spec _____
14. $\bar{c}$ _____
15. $\bar{\bar{s}}$ _____
16. $\bar{s}$ _____
17. pt _____
18. BP _____
19. R _____
20. Na _____
21. CDC _____
22. DRG _____
23. LMP _____

24. ♂ _____

25. ♀ _____

B. Look up the meanings of the following combinations to interpret the orders. Print your answers.

1. TPR qid _____
_____

2. 2 gtts bid _____
_____

3. 1 cc IM _____
_____

4. BP q 4 h _____
_____

5. 2 oz OJ qid ac and HS _____
_____

6. Wt and Ht qod in AM _____
_____

7. BR c̄ BRP only _____
_____

8. 1000 cc N/S IV _____
_____

9. Do ECG in CCU _____
_____

10. Dissolve 2 tsp NaCl in 1 qt H_2O _____
_____

11. 1000 cc SSE at HS _____
_____

12. Schedule B1 Wk in AM including CBC, BUN, and FBS _____
_____

13. Dilute 1 tab in 1 pt H_2O _____
_____

14. 1 cap qid pc and HS _____
_____

15. BP is measured in mm of Hg _____
_____

16. NPO pre-op _____
_____

17. Do EENT exam in OPD _____
_____

18. Ob-Gyn _____

_____

19. 500 mg qod 8 AM _____

_____

20. VS stat and q2h _____

_____

21. To PT by w/c for ROMs and ADL bid _____

_____

22. FF1 cl liq to 240 cc q2h _____

_____

23. 2 gtts OU qid q6h _____

_____

24. Dx: COPD, O_{12} prn, IPPB bid q12h _____

_____

25. Sig: $\ddot{\pi}$ Cap po tid $\bar{c}$ food or milk _____

_____

Name _____ Date _____

Evaluated by _____

DIRECTIONS: Read the case history aloud, using words instead of the abbreviations. Each abbreviation has a value of 5 points.

PROFICIENT

Using Medical Abbreviations	Points Possible	Peer Check		Final Check*		Points Earned**	Comments
		Yes	No	Yes	No		
1. Mary was taking medicine *ac* because the *Dr* ordered it. She was complaining of not feeling well so the orders included tests to find out the reason: a *CBC* was done and also a *FBS*. When he received the results, Dr. Pierce made a *dx* of diabetes and asked the *RN* to give Mary insulin. Mary now has to take insulin *qd* by *sc inj* and is on a *low cal* diet.	45						
2. A man was brought into the *ER* but he was *DOA*. The ambulance attendant said that the man had complained of headache, his *BP* was very high, and he may have had a *CVA*.	20						
3. John Smith was taken to the *Orth Dept* after a fall. He had a *Fr* of the knee that required surgery. After going to the *OR*, John was given medication *prn* for pain and was scheduled for *PT* to start next week for *ROM* exercises and *ADL*.	35						
Totals	100						

* Final Check: Instructor or authorized person evaluates.
** Points Earned: Points possible times each "yes" check.

CHAPTER 5:2 INTERPRETING WORD PARTS

ASSIGNMENT SHEET

Grade _____ Name _____

INTRODUCTION: Special words used in medicine are called medical terminology. Many of these words have common beginnings (prefixes), common endings (suffixes), and common parts (word roots). By learning the main prefixes, suffixes, and word roots, it is possible to put together many new words or to break apart a medical term to understand its meaning.

In the health fields, you will be required to know and understand medical terminology. Even if you have never come into contact with a medical word before, by breaking it down into its parts, you will usually be able to figure out the meaning of the word. This assignment sheet will show you the process.

INSTRUCTIONS: Review the information sheet on prefixes, suffixes, and word roots.

Study the following examples of breaking a word into parts.

Example 1: *erythrocyte:* erythro / cyte

      erythro means red

      cyte means cell

      erythrocyte means red cell

Example 2: *hyperadenosis:* hyper / aden / osis

      hyper means increased

      aden means gland

      osis means condition, state, or process

      hyperadenosis means increased glandular condition

A. **Identifying Word Parts:** Determine the meanings of the following words. Print your answers in the spaces provided. The words have been separated to help you do this exercise.

  1. crani / otomy _____

     crani _____

     otomy _____

  2. dys / uria _____

     dys _____

     uria _____

  3. hyster / ectomy _____

     hyster _____

     ectomy _____

  4. hemo / toxic _____

     hemo _____

     toxic _____

5. peri / card / itis _____

   peri _____

   card _____

   itis _____

6. leuko / cyte _____

   leuko _____

   cyte _____

7. chole / cyst / itis _____

   chole _____

   cyst _____

   itis _____

8. tachy / cardia _____

   tachy _____

   cardia _____

9. neur / algia _____

   neur _____

   algia _____

10. poly / cyt / emia _____

    poly _____

    cyt _____

    emia _____

11. brady / cardia _____

    _____

    _____

12. gastr / ectomy _____

    _____

    _____

13. mening / itis _____

    _____

    _____

14. neo / pathy _____

    _____

    _____

15. dermat / ologist _____

    _____

    _____

16. procto / scope _____

    _____

    _____

17. carcin / oma _____

_____

_____

18. electro / encephalo / graph _____

_____

_____

_____

19. osteo / malacia _____

_____

_____

20. para / plegia _____

_____

_____

21. py / uria _____

_____

_____

22. acro / megaly _____

_____

_____

23. geront / ology _____

_____

_____

24. dys / phagia _____

_____

_____

25. hydro / cele _____

_____

_____

B. Analyzing Words: Analyze each word to determine the breaking-off point. Mentally separate them into word elements. Print the meaning of the word.

1. adenoma _____

_____

_____

2. antitoxic _____

_____

_____

3. ophthalmology _____

_____

_____

4. cholecystectomy _____

_____

_____

5. endocarditis _____

_____

_____

6. gastroenteritis _____

_____

_____

7. hypoglycemia _____

_____

_____

8. septicemia _____

_____

_____

9. oliguria _____

_____

_____

10. bronchitis _____

_____

_____

11. homogeneous _____

_____

_____

12. arteriosclerosis _____

_____

_____

13. dysmenorrhea _____

_____

_____

14. angiopathy _____

_____

_____

15. blepharorrhaphy _____

_____

_____

16. urethrocystitis _____

_____

_____

17. pneumonomelanosis _____

_____

_____

18. paraosteoarthropathy _____

_____

_____

19. salpingo-oophorocele _____

_____

_____

20. idiopathic thrombocytopenia _____

_____

_____

21. narcoepilepsy _____

_____

_____

22. postpartum _____

_____

_____

23. herniorrhaphy _____

_____

_____

24. dermacyanosis _____

_____

_____

25. thoracentesis _____

_____

_____

Name _____ Date _____

Evaluated by _____

DIRECTIONS: Be able to tell your instructor the meaning of the *italicized words.* Pronunciation, spelling, and definition of the medical term will be evaluated. Be prepared to spell the word without looking at the term.

PROFICIENT

Prefixes, Suffixes, and Word Roots	Points Possible	Peer Check Yes	No	Final Check* Yes	No	Points Earned**	Comments
1. Mary had *dermalgia* that was caused by a rash.	10						
2. Mary's friend had *thrombophlebitis.*	10						
3. *Anuria* may be a sign of kidney disease.	10						
4. A *nephrectomy* requires a surgeon's skill.	10						
5. The *gastric* secretions were high in acid content.	10						
6. A *hysterectomy* was done to remove the tumor.	10						
7. *Hyperglycemia* may be a sign of diabetes.	10						
8. *Cholecystitis* may be caused by eating large quantities of undigestible fats.	10						
9. A fractured neck can cause *quadriplegia.*	10						
10. *Hepatitis* can produce a yellow tinge to the skin.	10						
Totals	100						

* Final Check: Instructor or authorized person evaluates.
** Points Earned: Points possible times each "yes" check.

ASSIGNMENT SHEET

Grade _____ Name _____

INTRODUCTION: A basic understanding of the structure of the human body will help a health care worker understand the total function of the body. This assignment will help you review the main facts.

INSTRUCTIONS: Read the information on Basic Structure of the Human Body. In the space provided, print the word(s) that best completes the statement or answers the question.

1. Label the parts of the cell on the following illustration. Briefly state the function of each part.

smooth endoplasmic reticulum B

nucleolus D

nucleus C

G mitochondrion

A cell membrane

pinocytic vessel J

F cytoplasm

lysosome I

Golgi apparatus H

E chromatin

A.   F.

B.   G.

C.   H.

D.   I.

E.   J.

2. The study of the form and structure of an organism is _anatomy_. The study of the processes of living organisms is _physiology_. The study of how disease occurs is _pathophysiology_.

3. What is the basic unit of structure and function in all living things?
   ~~Protoplasm~~ Cell

4. List four (4) functions of cells.
   - take in food & oxygen
   - produce heat & energy
   - move & adapt to their enviroment
   - eliminate wastes

5. What is the form of asexual reproduction used by cells?
   Mitosis

   Briefly sketch this process and state what occurs in each step.

   ① DNA molecules duplicate themselves

   ② Centrioles separate & spindles form between them

   ③ Duplicated Chromosomes line up along center of spindle

   ④ Chromosomes seperate

   ⑤ Two nuclei form as cell seperates

   ⑥ Each new cell has the same number of chromosomes

6. What condition results from an insufficient amount of tissue fluid?
   Dehydration

   What condition results from an excess amount of tissue fluid?
   Edema

7. List the four (4) main types of tissues and state the function of each type.
   1) Epithelial Tissue- covers the surface of the body & is the main Tissue
   2) Connective Tissue- the supporting fabric of organs & other body parts
   3) Nerve Tissue- made up of special cells call neurons, controls & coordinates body activities
   4) Muscle Tissue- produces power & movement by contraction of muscle fibers

8. What is the proper name for fatty tissue?

Adipose tissue

List three (3) functions of fatty tissue.
- Stores fat as a food reserve or source of energy
- insulates the body
- acts as padding

9. How does bone tissue differ from cartilage?

Cartilage - a tough, elastic material found between the bones of the spine + at the end of the long bones
Bone Tissue - similar to cartilage but has calcium salts, nerves, + blood vessels

10. List the three (3) main types of muscle tissue and state the function of each type.
1) Skeletal - attaches the bones + provides for movement for the body
2) Cardiac - causes the heart to beat
3) Visceral - present in the walls of the digestive tract

11. When two or more tissues join together for a specific function, they form a/an
stomach ____~~System~~ organ____. Examples include ____~~Muscular~~ heart____,
~~muscle~~ ____~~Circulatory~~____, and ____~~Skeletal~~ lungs____

12. Name ten (10) body systems.

1) reproductive   6) lymphatic
2) endocrine   7) circulatory
3) urinary   8) nervous
4) digestive   9) muscular
5) respiratory   10) skeletal

CHAPTER 6:2 BODY PLANES, DIRECTIONS, AND CAVITIES

ASSIGNMENT SHEET

Grade _____ Name _____

INTRODUCTION: Directional terms are used to describe the relationship of one part of the body to another part. This assignment will help you review the main terms used.

INSTRUCTIONS: Read the information on Body Planes, Directions, and Cavities. In the space provided, print the word(s) that best completes the statement or answers the question.

1. Place the letter of the correct term in Column B in the space provided by a description of the term in Column A.

	Column A	**Column B**
1. _C_	Body parts away from the point of reference	A. Caudal
2. _L_	Horizontal plane that divides the body into a top and bottom half	B. Cranial
3. _G_	Body parts away from the midline	C. Distal
4. _F_	Body parts below the transverse plane	D. Dorsal or posterior
5. _M_	Body parts on the front of the body	E. Frontal
6. _I_	Plane that divides the body into a right and left side	F. Inferior
7. _J_	Body parts close to the point of reference	G. Lateral
8. _B_	Body parts located near the head	H. Medial
9. _K_	Body parts above the transverse plane	I. Midsaggital
10. _D_	Body parts on the back of the body	J. Proximal
11. _H_	Body parts close to the midline	K. Superior
12. _A_	Body parts located near sacral region or "tail"	L. Transverse
13. _E_	Plane that divides body into front and back section	M. Ventral or anterior

2. Identify the body cavities in the following illustration.

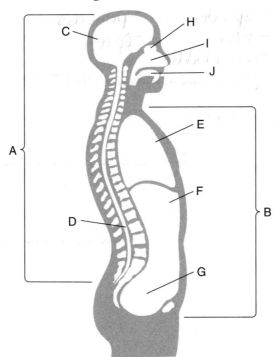

A. ~~Spinal (vertebral canal)~~ Dorsal cavity
B. Ventral cavity
C. Crainal cavity
D. Spinal (vertebral canal)
E. Thoracic cavity
F. Abdominal cavity
G. Pelvic cavity
H. orbital cavity
I. nasal cavity
J. buccal cavity

3. List the organs located in each of the following body cavities.

cranial:
 - the brain
 - the spinal cavity (contains the spinal cord)

spinal:
 - spinal cord

thoracic:
 - esophagus   - lungs
 - trachea   - heart
 - bronchi   - large blood vessels

upper abdominal:
- Stomach   - appendex   - pancreas
- small intestine - liver   - spleen
- most of the   - gall bladder
  large intestine
pelvic: (lower abdominal)
- urinary bladder
- reproductive organs
- last part of the
  large intestine
orbital:
- eyes

nasal:
- nose structures

buccal: (mouth)
- teeth
- toungue

4. The abdominal cavity can be divided into quadrants or four (4) main sections. Name these sections and the proper abbreviation for each section.

1) Right Upper Quadrant = RUQ
2) left Upper Quadrant = LUQ
3) Right lower Quadrant = RLQ
4) left lower Quadrant = LLQ

5. Identify the abdominal region for each of the following descriptions.

epigastric   a. ~~left upper quad.~~   region above the stomach
right iliac region b. ~~left lower quad.~~   region on the right side by the groin
~~left lumbar reg.~~ c. ~~right lower quad.~~ hypocondriac region on the left side below the ribs
umbilical reg. d. ~~all four~~   region by the umbilicus or belly-button
↓ lumbar   e. ~~left upper + lower~~   region on the right side by the large bones of the spinal cord
pelvic   f. ~~left lower quad~~   region below the stomach
                   hypogastric

CHAPTER 6:3 INTEGUMENTARY SYSTEM

ASSIGNMENT SHEET

Grade _____   Name _____

INTRODUCTION: The integumentary system consists of the skin and all its parts. This assignment will help you review the main facts of this system.

INSTRUCTIONS: Read the information on the Integumentary System. In the space provided, print the word(s) that best completes the statement or answers the question.

1. Label the following diagram of a cross-section of the skin.

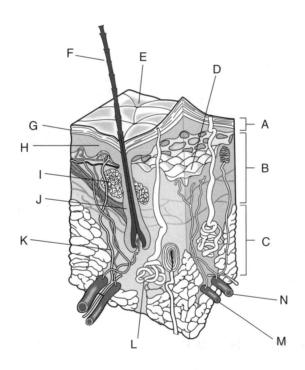

A. Epidermis

B. Dermis

C. Subcutaneous

D. Dermal Papilla

E. Sweat Pore

F. Hair Shaft

G. Stratum Corneum

H. Stratum Spinosum

I. Sebaceous (oil) gland

J. Hair Follicle

K. Nerve Fiber

L. Sweat Gland

M. Artery

N. Vein

2. What are papillae?

   Ridges on the hand.

   How do they provide a method of identification?

   They make up your fingerprints.

3. What is the proper name for sweat glands?

   Sudoriferous glands

   Name three (3) substances found in perspiration.
   - *water*
   - *salts*
   - *some body wastes*

4. What is the proper name for oil glands?

   Sebaceous Glands

   What are the functions of oil glands?

   They produce sebum, an oil that helps skin and hair from becoming dry + brittle.

5. What is alopecia?

   Baldness.

6. List seven (7) functions of the skin.

   1) *Protection*
   2) *Sensory Perception*
   3) *Body temperature regulation*
   4) *Storage*
   5) *Absorption*
   6) *excretion*
   7) *production*

7. What happens when blood vessels dilate? How does this regulate temperature?

   Excess heat from the blood vessels can escape through the skin. It helps the body retain/lose heat.

   What happens when blood vessels constrict? How does this regulate temperature?

   The heat is retained in the body. This helps retain/lose heat.

8. Define the following words, and give one cause for each discoloration.

   a. erythema: *A reddish color of the skin caused by burns or a congestion of the blood vessels*

   b. jaundice: *A yellow discoloration of the skin caused by liver/gallbladder disease*

   c. cyanosis: *A bluish discoloration of the skin caused by insufficient oxygen*

9. Identify the following skin eruptions.

   a. blisters or sacs full of fluid: Vesicles

   b. firm raised areas on the skin: Papules

   c. areas of dried pus and blood: Crusts

   d. sacs filled with pus: Pustules

   e. flat spots on the skin: Macules

   f. itchy, elevated areas with an irregular shape: Wheals

   g. deep loss of skin surface that may extend into dermis: Ulcer

10. Briefly describe the following skin diseases.

   a. impetigo: highly contagious skin infection usually caused by streptococci or staphylococci organisms. Symptoms are erythema, oozing vesicles, pustules, & the formation of a yellow crust

   b. verrucae: warts caused by a viral infection of the skin. A rough, hard, elevated, rounded surface forms on the skin.

   c. dermatitis: An inflamation of the skin caused by any substance that irritates the skin. Frequently an allergic reaction to detergents, cosmetics, pollen, or certain foods. Symptoms include dry skin, erythema, itching, edema, macular-papular rashes, & scaling.

   d. acne vulgaris: An inflamation of the sebaceous glands. The cause is unknown. Symptoms include papules, pustules, & blackheads.

   e. athlete's foot: A contagious fungal infection that usually affects the feet. The skin itches, and blisters and cracks into open sores. Treatment involves applying an antifungal medication & keeping the area dry & clean.

   f. psoriasis: A chronic, noncontagious, inherited skin disease. Symptoms include thick red areas covered with white or silver scales. There isn't a cure.

   g. ringworm: A highly contagious fungus infection of the skin or scalp. The symptom is the formation of a flat or raised circular area with a clear central area surrounded by an itchy, scaly, or crusty outer ring. Antifungal treatments are used.

ASSIGNMENT SHEET

Grade _____   Name _____

INTRODUCTION: The skeletal system forms the framework of the entire body. This assignment will help you review the main facts about this system.

INSTRUCTIONS: Read the information on the Skeletal System. In the space provided, print the word(s) that best completes the statement or answers the question.

1. Use the Key Terms to complete the following crossword puzzle.

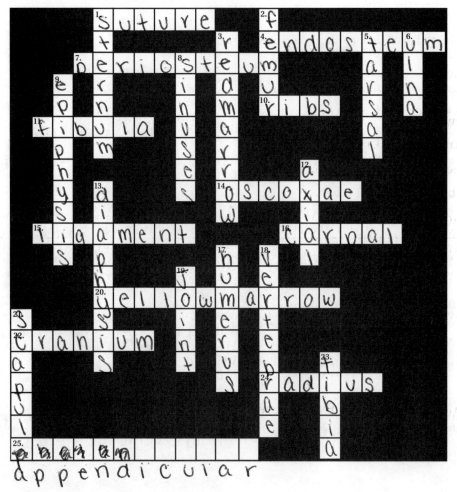

appendicular

ACROSS

1. Area where cranial bones have joined together

4. Membrane that lines the medullary canal

7. Tough membrane on the outside of bone

10. Twelve pairs of bones that surround the heart and lungs

11. Lateral bone of the lower leg

14. Two bones that form the pelvic girdle

15. Connective tissue band that holds bones together

16. Wrist bone

20. Material inside the medullary canal

22. Eight bones that surround and protect the brain

24. Lower arm bone on thumb side

✗ 25. Bones that form the extremities

DOWN

1. Breastbone

2. Thigh bone

3. Material found in some bones that produces blood cells

5. Anklebone

6. Larger bone of lower arm

✗ 8. Air spaces in the bones of the skull

9. An extremity or end of bone

12. Bones that form the main trunk of the body

13. Long shaft of bones

17. Upper arm bone

18. Twenty-six bones of the spinal column

19. Area where two or more bones join together

21. Shoulder bone or shoulder blade

23. Medial bone of the lower leg

2. List five (5) functions of bones.
   1) framework
   2) protection
   3) levers
   4) production of blood cells
   5) storage

3. Name the eight (8) bones that form the cranium.
   - one frontal   - one ethimoid
   - two parietal   - one sphenoid
   - two temperol
   - one occipital

4. Name the twenty-six (26) vertebrae.
   - 7 cervical
   - 12 thoracic
   - 5 lumbar
   - 1 sacrum
   - coccyx

5. What is the difference between true ribs, false ribs, and floating ribs?

—true: 1st 7 pair, attach to the ~~thoracic vertebrae~~ sternum
- False: next 5, first 3 pairs attach to cartilage
- floating: last 2 pairs of false, have no attatchment on the front of the body

6. What is the name of the small piece of cartilage at the bottom of the sternum?
   - Xiphoid process

7. What are the three (3) regions on each os coxae?
   - Samphysis pops   - ilium
   - acetabula   - ishium
   - Obturator foramen   - pubis

8. Name the three (3) main types of joints. Describe the degree of movement, and give an example for each type.
   - Diarthrosis: ball + socket joints
   - amphiarthrosis: ribs attatched to thoracic vertebrae
   - Synarthrosis: cranium

9. What is the purpose of ligaments?
   - help hold long bones together at joints

10. Briefly describe the following diseases or disorders of the skeletal system.
    a. arthritis: inflamation of the joints

    b. fractures: crack/break in the bone

    c. osteomyelitis: bone inflamation usually caused by a pathogenic organism

    d. osteoporosis: softening of the bones

    e. sprain: twisting action tears the legiments at a joint

    f. bursitis: inflamation of the fluid-filled sacs around the joints

    g. dislocation: when a bone is forcibly displaced from a joint

    h. scoliosis: abnormal curvatures of the spinal column

Name _____

11. Label the skeleton with the correct names for all the bones.

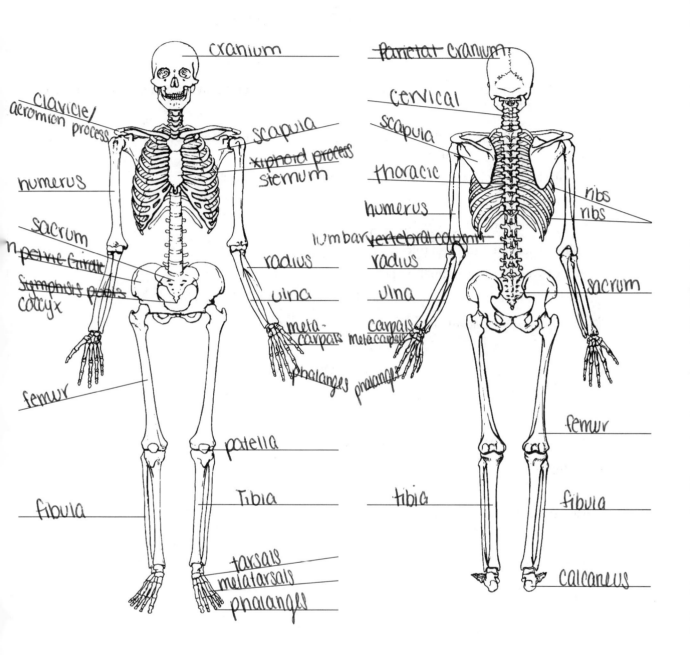

cranium

Parietal cranium

clavicle/ acromion process

cervical

scapula

scapula

humerus

xiphoid process sternum

thoracic

sacrum

humerus

n pelvic Girdle

lumbar vertebral column

Symphsis pubis

radius

radius

coccyx

ulna

ulna

meta- carpals

carpals metacarpals

sacrum

femur

phalanges phalanges

patella

femur

Tibia

tibia

fibula

fibula

fibula

tarsals

metatarsals

phalanges

calcaneus

CHAPTER 6:5 MUSCULAR SYSTEM

ASSIGNMENT SHEET

Grade _____ Name _____

INTRODUCTION: The muscular system provides movement for the body. This assignment will help you review the main facts about this system.

INSTRUCTIONS: Read the information on the Muscular System. In the space provided, print the word(s) that best completes the statement or answers the question.

1. Identify each of the following properties or characteristics of muscles.

    a. ability to respond to a stimulus: excitability

    b. ability to be stretched: extensibility

    c. ability to become short and thick: contractibility

    d. ability to return to its original shape: elasticity

2. List the three (3) main kinds of muscles and the main function of each kind.
    - cardiac- lines the walls of the heart
    - visceral- internal organs
    - skeletal- attached to bones + causes movement

3. What is the difference between voluntary and involuntary muscles?
    - voluntary- have control
    - involuntary- don't have control

4. List four (4) functions of skeletal muscles.
    - provide voluntary movement
    - produce heat + energy
    - help maintain posture
    - protect internal organs

5. Name two (2) ways skeletal muscles attach to bones.
    - tendons
    - fascia

6. Identify the following action or movement performed by muscles.

    a. decreasing the angle between two bones: flexion

    b. swinging the arm around in a circle: circumduction

    c. moving a body part toward the midline: adduction

    d. bending the lower arm up towards the upper arm: flexion

    e. moving the arm away from the side of the body: abduction

    f. straightening the lower leg away from the upper leg: extension

    g. increasing the angle between two bones: extension

    h. turning a body part on its own axis: rotation

    i. moving the leg in toward the body: adduction

    j. turning the head from side to side: rotation

7. What is muscle tone?

partial contraction of a muscle

8. What occurs when muscles atrophy? What causes muscles to atrophy?

- shrink in size + lose strength
- muscles aren't used for a long period of time

9. What is a contracture?

a severe tightening of a flexor muscle

Name the joints affected most frequently by contractures.

- foot   - wrists
- fingers   - knees

10. Name the following muscles.

   a. muscle of upper arm that flexes lower arm: *biceps brachii*

   b. muscle on front of thigh that abducts and flexes leg: *rectus femoris sartorius*

   c. muscle on upper back and neck that extends head and moves shoulder: *trapezius*

   d. muscles between ribs used for breathing: *intercostals*

   e. muscle on front of lower leg that flexes and inverts the foot: *tibialis anterior*

   f. two muscles that can be used as injection sites: *deltoid, gluteus maximus*

   g. muscle that compresses the abdomen: *rectus abdominus*

   h. muscle on upper chest that adducts upper arm: *pectoralis major*

   i. muscle on side of neck that turns and flexes head: *sternocleidomastoid*

   j. muscle on front of thigh that extends leg: *quadriceps femoris*

11. Unscramble the following words to identify some diseases of the muscular system. Then give a brief description of each disease.

   a. LUMCSE PASMSS:
   muscle spasms
   - cramps
   - muscle contractions

   b. CASMULRU PTSDOHYRY:
   muscular dystrophy
   - inherited

   c. YAHMTNSIEA RVGISA:
   myasthenia gravis
   - nerve impulses not transmitted to muscles

   d. RISATN:
   strain

   e. GIBOYLFIRAMA:
   fibromyalgia
   - chronic
   - wide spread
   - pain in muscle sites

CHAPTER 6:6 NERVOUS SYSTEM

ASSIGNMENT SHEET

Grade _____ Name _____

INTRODUCTION: The nervous system coordinates all the activities of the body. This assignment will help you review the main facts about this system.

INSTRUCTIONS: Read the information on the Nervous System. In the space provided, print the word(s) that best completes the statement or answers the question.

1. Some of the Key Terms are hidden in the following puzzle. Can you find the following terms?

autonomic nervous system

brain

central nervous system

cerebellum

cerebrospinal fluid

cerebrum

medulla oblongata

meninge

midbrain

nerve

neuron

parasympathetic

peripheral nervous system

pons

spinal cord

sympathetic

ventricle

```
S E T P A R A S Y M P A T H E T I C M I U B E M S D
A V N E M R U R E N T H E C M R S E D T I C E I L W
T X Q R Z D E I U T E L C I R T N E V X L O V D E S
A I D I U L F L A N I P S O R B E R E C M M E B R F
G L O P Y D J O S E S H A R O L U O U I S E X R W T
N A N H N I A M A R K A R E C E R E B R U M C A E R
O E C E R E B E L L U M B R U M O S Y S T O M I T H
L I S R I S C R A Z E N A N D I N A M N O T S N U R
B E W A H Y I A M D O E I M G I D R O C L A N I P S
O T B L U T Y G U E S R S H A V U N R I C T K E O X
A C E N T R A L N E R V O U S S Y S T E M W O G N U
L L D E U N D E R B L E O O D L Y M P H E R Y N S P
L S B R A I N P I C I T E H T A P M Y S N A L I C O
U R D V N A T O P H Y S I O L E G E E R T S D N M I
D D I O V E R S I O C C F E D I P A Y T I O N E L J
E X A U T O N O M I C N E R V O U S S Y S T E M M H
M C A S Y S T E M N Y O U F I N D T H E W O R D S I
```

2. The basic structural unit of the nervous system is the __neuron__. It consists of a cell body that contains the __nucleus__, nerve fibers called __dendrites__, which carry impulses toward the cell body, and a single nerve fiber called a/an __axon__, which carries impulses away from the cell body. Many axons have a lipid covering called a/an __myelin sheath__, which increases the rate of transmission of a/an __impulse__, and __insulates__ and __maintains__ the axon.

3. What is a synapse?

   The space between ~~axons~~ dendrites.

4. Identify all the parts of the brain shown on the diagram. Briefly state the function of each part.

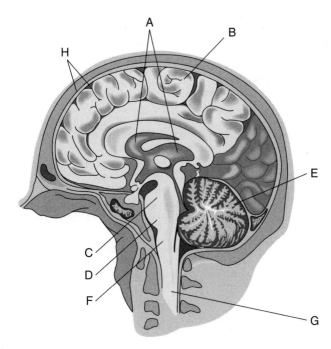

cerebrum

A. lateral ventricle - hollow spaces, contain CSF

B. convolutions - wrinkles; help increase memory

C. midbrain - reflect actions of the eye

D. pons - respiration, chewing, tasting

E. cerebellum - balance

F. medulla oblongata - respiration, heart beat

G. spinal cord - reflex actions

H. sulci

5. Name the three (3) layers of the meninges.

1) dura mater
2) arachnoid membrane
3) pia mater

What is the function of the meninges?

To cover/protect the brain and spinal cord.

6. List two (2) functions of cerebrospinal fluid.
- shock absorber
- carries nutrients

7. The peripheral nervous system consists of the __somatic__ and the __autonomic__ nervous systems. The somatic nervous system consists of 12 pairs of __cranial nerves__ and 31 pairs of __spinal nerves__.

8. State the actions that the sympathetic and parasympathetic nervous systems have on the following functions of the body.

	Sympathetic	Parasympathetic
heart rate	increase	slow
respirations	increase	decrease
blood pressure	increase	lower
digestive activity	slow activity	increase

9. What is homeostasis?

A balanced state of the body.

10. Briefly describe the following diseases of the nervous system.

a. paraplegia: paralysis in the lower extremities; caused by a spinal cord injury

b. encephalitis: inflamation of the brain

c. hydrocephalus: excessive accumulation of cerebrospinal fluid in the ventricles

d. neuralgia: nerve pain

e. cerebrovascular accident: stroke; when the blood flow to the brain is impaired

f. epilepsy: seizure

g. cerebral palsy: disturbance in voluntary muscle action

h. Parkinson's disease: degeneration of the brain cells

CHAPTER 6:7 SPECIAL SENSES

ASSIGNMENT SHEET

Grade _____ Name _____

INTRODUCTION: Special senses allow the human body to react to the environment. This assignment will help you review the main facts about these senses.

INSTRUCTIONS: Read the information on Special Senses. In the space provided, print the word(s) that best completes the statement or answers the question.

1. Special senses occur because the body has organs that receive ___sensation___, nerves that carry the message to the ___brain___, and a brain that ___interprets___ and ___responds___ to the message.

2. Label the following diagram of the eye and briefly state the function of each part.

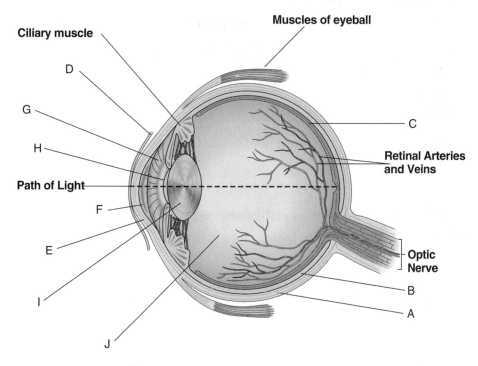

A. Sclera - outer protection
B. Choroid coat - nourishes
C. retina
D. conjunctiva
E. cornea

F. ~~has~~ Anterior chamber
G. iris
H. pupil
I. lens
J. Posterior chamber

3. List four (4) structures that protect the eye.
   - socket
   - eyelids
   - eyelashes
   - tear ducts

4. Name five (5) parts of the eye that light rays pass through to focus on the retina.
   - cornea   - lens
   - aqueous humor   - vitreous humor
   - pupil

   What happens if these parts do not refract the light rays correctly?
   Vision can be distorted
   or blurred.

5. Name the following eye diseases.

   a. an abnormal shape or curvature in the cornea that causes blurred vision: estigmatism

   b. increased intraocular pressure caused by an excess amount of aqueous humor: glaucoma

   c. nearsightedness: myopia

   d. crossed eyes resulting from a weakness in eye muscles: strabismus

   e. lens become cloudy or opaque: cataract

   f. contagious inflammation of conjunctiva: conjunctivitis

   g. farsightedness caused by a loss of elasticity in the lens: presbyopia

6. What is cerumen? What is its function?
   - wax plug
   - foreign body obstruction
   - protects the ear

7. What is the correct name for the eardrum? What does it do?
   - Tympanic membrane
   - separates the outer ear from
   the inner ear

8. Name the three (3) bones or ossicles of the middle ear.
   - malleus
   - incus
   - stapes

9. What is the eustachian tube? What does it do?
   - tube that connects the middle ear to the throat
   - equilizes air pressure

10. State the function of the following parts of the inner ear.

    a. vestibule: entrance to 2 other parts of the inner ear

    b. cochlea: contains hairlike cells

    c. organ of Corti: receptor of sound waves

    d. semicircular canals: help to maintain a sense of balance

11. An infection of the middle ear is _Otitis media_. A hearing loss caused by lack of movement of the stapes is _Otosclerosis_____. If sound waves are not being conducted to the inner ear, this causes a/an _Conductive_____ hearing loss or deafness. Damage to the inner ear or auditory nerve causes a/an _Sensory_____ hearing loss or deafness.

12. List the four (4) main tastes. Where are they located on the tongue?
    - sweet: tip of the tounge
    - salty: tip of the tounge
    - sour: side
    - bitter: back

13. What determines the sense of smell?
    olefactory receptors

14. Name four (4) general sense receptors located throughout the body.
    - pressure
    - heat/cold
    - touch
    - pain

ASSIGNMENT SHEET

Grade _____   Name _____

INTRODUCTION: The circulatory system is often called the transportation system of the body. This assignment will help you review the main facts on this system.

INSTRUCTIONS: Read the information on the Circulatory System. In the space provided, print the word(s) that best answers the question or completes the statement.

1. Use the Key Terms to complete the crossword puzzle.

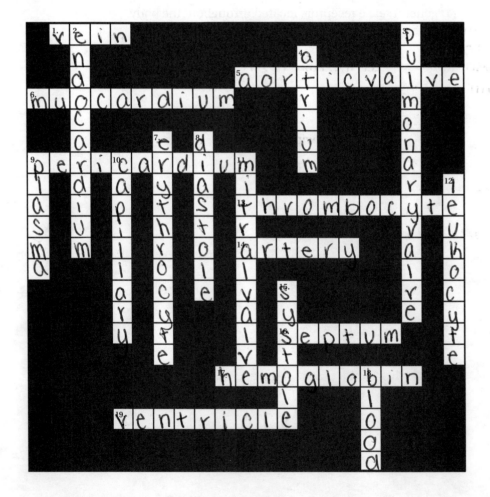

ACROSS

1. Blood vessel that carries blood back to the heart
5. Valve between the left ventricle and aorta
6. Muscular middle layer of the heart
9. Double-layered membrane on the outside of the heart
13. Blood cell required for the clotting process
14. Blood vessel that carries blood away from the heart
16. Muscular wall that separates the heart into a right and left side
17. Complex protein on red blood cells
19. Lower chamber of the heart

DOWN

2. Smooth layer of cells lining the inside of the heart
3. Valve between the right ventricle and pulmonary artery
4. Upper chamber of the heart
7. Blood cell that carries oxygen and carbon dioxide
8. Brief period of rest in the heart
9. Fluid portion of blood
10. Blood vessel that connects arterioles with venules
11. Valve between the left atrium and left ventricle
12. Blood cell that helps fight infection
15. Period of ventricular contraction in the heart
18. Tissue that flows through the circulatory system

2. Label the following diagram of the heart.

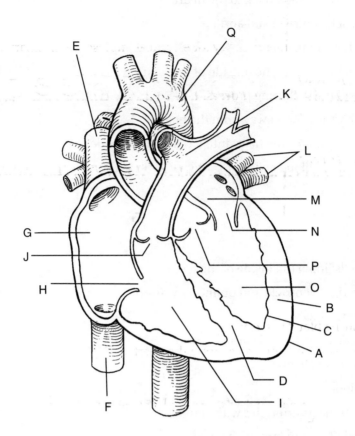

A. Pericardium

B. Myocardium

C. Endocardium

D. Septum

E. Superior Vena Cava

F. Inferior Vena Cava

G. Right Atrium

H. Tricuspid valve

I. Right Ventricle

J. Pulmonary Semilunar Valve

K. Pulmonary Artery

L. Pulmonary Veins

M. Left Atrium

N. Bicuspid Valve

O. Left Ventricle

P. Aortic Semilunar Valve

Q. Aorta

3. Describe what happens in the heart during diastole.

During Diastole the heart relaxes and allows blood returning from the body to enter into the right atrium while blood returning from the lungs enters the left atrium.

Name _____

4. Describe what happens in the heart during systole. State where each ventricle sends the blood.
During systole the ventricles contract which allows for the right ventricle to push blood into the pulmonary artery to the lungs, and the left pushes blood to the aorta to be distributed throughout the body.

5. List the parts of the conductive pathway for electrical impulses in the heart. List the parts in correct order.
Heart - Sinoatrial node - atria muscles - ventricles - atrioventricular node - bundle of His - right/left bundle branches - Purkinje Fibers

6. What is arrhythmia? How is it diagnosed?
Arrythmia is an abnormal heart rythm that can be mild to life-threatening. They are diagnosed by cardiac moniters and electrocardiograms.

7. Identify the following blood vessels:
   a. blood vessels that carry blood away from the heart: Arteries
   b. blood vessels that carry blood back to the heart: Veins
   c. blood vessels that connect arterioles with venules: Capillaries
   d. largest artery in the body: Aorta
   e. two largest veins in the body: Superior/Inferior Vena Cava
   f. vessels that allow oxygen and nutrients to pass through to cells: Capillaries
   g. smallest branches of arteries: Arterioles
   h. smallest branches of veins: Venules
   i. vessels that contain valves to prevent backflow of blood: Veins
   j. most muscular and elastic blood vessels: Arteries

8. List six (6) substances transported by the blood.
   - Oxygen   - metabolic/waste products
   - Carbon dioxide   - heat
   - nutrients   - hormones

9. List six (6) substances that are dissolved or suspended in plasma.
   - blood protiens   - gases
   - nutrients
   - mineral salts/   - metabolic/waste products
     electrolytes
                           - hormones/enzymes

10. Name the three (3) main types of blood cells. State the normal count and the function of each type.

Blood Cell	Normal Count Per Cubic Millimeter of Blood	Function
Erythrocytes	(Twenty-Five Trillion) 4.5-5.5 million per cmm	contains hemoglobin
leukocytes	5,000-10,000 per cmm	fight infection
Thrombocytes	250,000-400,000 per cmm	clotting process

11. What gives blood its characteristic red color?
Hemoglobin that carries a lot of oxygen.

12. What is hemoglobin? What is its function?
A complex protein composed of a protein molecule called globin and the iron compound called heme.

13. Identify the type of leukocyte(s) that performs the following function.

a. phagocytize bacteria: Neutrophils ~~Lymphocytes~~ Monocytes

b. provide immunity for the body by developing antibodies: Lymphocytes

c. defend the body from allergic reactions: Eosinophils

d. produce histamine and heparin: Basophils

14. Name the following diseases of the circulatory system.

a. saclike formation in the wall of an artery: Aneurysm

b. inadequate number of red blood cells, hemoglobin, or both: Pernicious anemia

c. dilated swollen veins: Varicose veins

d. a fatty deposit on the walls of arteries: Atherosclerosis

e. disease characterized by failure of the blood to clot: Hemophelia

f. high blood pressure: Hypertension

g. inflammation of the veins with formation of a clot: Thrombo-Phlebitis

h. blockage in the coronary arteries of the heart: Myocardial Infarction

i. foreign substance circulating in the blood stream: Embolus

j. malignant disease with large numbers of immature white blood cells: Leuhemia

CHAPTER 6:9 LYMPHATIC SYSTEM

ASSIGNMENT SHEET

Grade _____ Name _____

INTRODUCTION: The lymphatic system works with the circulatory system to remove waste and excess fluid from the tissues. This assignment will help you review the main facts about this system.

INSTRUCTIONS: Read the information on the Lymphatic System. In the space provided, print the word(s) that best completes the statement or answers the question.

1. What is lymph? Of what is it composed?

   It's a thin, watery fluid composed of intercellular (interstitial) fluid.

2. Small, open-ended lymph vessels called *lymphatic capillaries* pick up *lymph* at tissues throughout the body. They join together to form larger *lymphatic vessels* which pass through *lymph nodes*.

3. What keeps the lymph flowing in a one-way direction while it is in the lymphatic vessels?

   Valves

4. What are lacteals? What do they do?

   They are specialized lymphatic capillaries that pick up digested fat/lipids.

5. Name four (4) substances that are filtered from the lymph while it is in lymph nodes.

   - Carbon   - pathogens
   - cancer cells   - dead blood cells

6. Name two (2) things produced by the lymph tissues in lymph nodes.

   - lymphocytes
   - antibodies

7. Name the two (2) lymphatic ducts and the areas of the body that they drain.

   1) Right lymphatic ducts - empties into the right subclavian vein
   2) Thoracic Duct - left subclavian vein

8. What is the cisterni chyli? Where is it located?

   It's an enlarged pouchlike structure located at the start of the thoracic duct.

9. The purified lymph, with lymphocytes and antibodies added, returns to the *bloodstream* when it leaves the lymphatic ducts. The right lymphatic duct empties the purified lymph into the *right subclavian vein*, and the thoracic duct empties into the *left subclavian vein*

10. List the three (3) types of tonsils and state where they are located.

1) Palatine - each side of the soft palate
2) Pharyngeal - in the nasopharynx
3) lingual - on the back of the toungue

11. List four (4) functions of the spleen.

1) produces leukocytes + antibodies
2) destroys old erythrocytes
3) stores erythrocytes to release into the bloodstream
4) filters metabolites and wastes from body tissue

12. What is the thymus? What happens to it at puberty?

It is a mass of lymph tissue located in the upper chest that wastes away after puberty.

13. Name the following diseases of the lymphatic system.

    a. inflammation or infection of the lymph nodes or glands: Adenitis

    b. chronic malignant condition with enlargement of lymph nodes: Hodghins disease

    c. enlargement of the spleen: Splenomegaly

    d. inflammation of the tonsils: Tonsillitis

    e. inflammation of lymphatic vessels: lymphangitis

ASSIGNMENT SHEET

Grade _____ Name _____

INTRODUCTION: The respiratory system is responsible for taking in oxygen and removing carbon dioxide from the body. This assignment will help you review the main facts about this system.

INSTRUCTIONS: Read the information on the Respiratory System. In the space provided, print the word(s) that best completes the statement or answers the question.

1. Label the following diagram of the respiratory system.

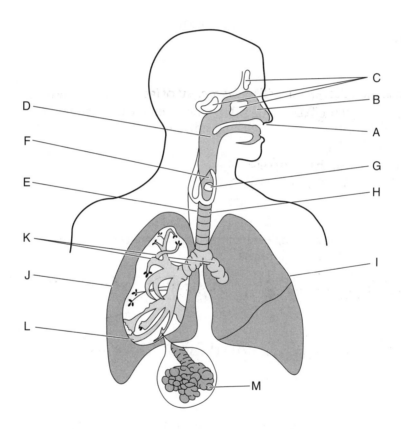

A. ~~oral cavity~~ nares

B. nasal cavity

C. sinuses

D. ~~larynx~~ pharynx

E. esophagus

F. ~~larynx~~ epiglottis

G. larynx

H. trachea

I. left lung

J. right lung

K. branchi

L. branchiole

M. alveoli

2. List three (3) things that happen to air when it enters the nasal cavity.
   - warmed
   - filtered
   - moistened

3. What are cilia? What do they do?
   - tiny, hairlike structures
   - help move the mucous ~~membrane~~ layer that lines the airways, pushing trapped particles toward the esophagus, where they can be swallowed

4. Name the three (3) sections of the pharynx.
   - nasopharynx: upper portion
   - oropharynx: middle section
   - laryngopharynx: bottom section

5. How is speech produced?
   The air leaving the lungs vibrates the vocal cords.

6. What prevents food and liquids from entering the respiratory tract?
   - epiglottis

7. The alveoli contains a rich network of blood capillaries They allow for the exchange of oxygen and carbon dioxide between the bloodstream and the lungs. The inner surfaces of the alveoli are covered with a lipid substance called surfacant to help prevent the alveoli from collapsing.

8. Why is the left lung smaller than the right lung?
   - the heart is located on the left

9. Describe what is happening during each of the following phases of respiration. Be sure to include the actions of the muscles during each phase.

   a. inspiration: breathing air. the diaphragm & intercostal muscles contract & enlarge the thoracic cavity to create a vacum

   b. expiration: exhalation; air is forced out of the lungs

10. How does external respiration differ from internal respiration?
    - external - exchange of CO_2 & O_2 between the lungs & bloodstream
    - internal - exchange of CO_2 & O_2 between the tissue cells & bloodstream

11. What is cellular respiration?
    When the cells use oxygen/nutrients to produce energy, water, & carbon dioxide.

12. What causes the respiratory center in the medulla oblongata of the brain to increase the rate of respirations?
    Increasing carbon dioxide

13. Use the names of respiratory diseases to fill in the blanks.

B R O N C H I T I S (inflammation of bronchi and bronchial tubes)

I N F L U E N Z A (highly contagious viral infection)

S I N U S I T I S (inflammation of mucous membrane lining sinuses)

E M P H Y S E M A (walls of alveoli deteriorate and lose their elasticity)

E P I S T A X I S (a nosebleed)

T U B E R C U L O S I S (infectious lung disease caused by bacteria)

A S T H M A (bronchospasms narrow the openings of the bronchioles)

R H I N I T I S (inflammation of nasal mucous membranes)

C O P D (any chronic lung disease that results in obstruction of the airways)

P L E U R I S Y (inflammation of membranes of the lungs)

L A R Y N G I T I S (inflammation of the voicebox and vocal cords)

14. A person you love is a heavy smoker. Briefly discuss at least four (4) respiratory diseases that are caused by smoking. Is there any way you can convince this person to quit smoking?

– lung cancer
– ~~pneumonia~~
– emphysema
– COPD
– bronchitis

CHAPTER 6:11 DIGESTIVE SYSTEM

ASSIGNMENT SHEET

Grade _____ Name _____

INTRODUCTION: The digestive system is responsible for the breakdown of food so it can be taken into the bloodstream and used by body cells and tissues. This assignment will help you review the main facts about this system.

INSTRUCTIONS: Read the information on the Digestive System. In the space provided, print the word(s) that best completes the statement or answers the question.

1. Label the diagram of the digestive system.

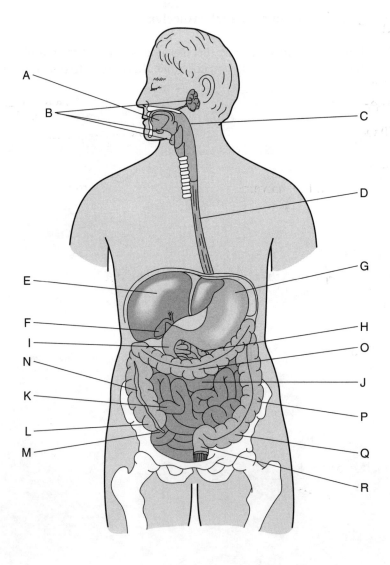

A. Tongue

B. Sublingual, parotid, + submandibular glands

C. pharynx

D. esophagus

E. liver

F. gallbladder

G. stomach

H. pancreas

I. duodenum

J. Jejunum

K. ileum

L. cecum

M. Vermiform appendix

N. ascending colon of large intestine

O. Transverse colon of the large intestine

P. descending colon of the large intestine

Q. sigmoid colon of the large intestine

R. rectum

2. List two (2) functions of the tongue.
   —taste buds allow for tasting of foods
   —aids in chewing/swallowing food

3. What is mastication?
   The breakdown of food by chewing and grinding with the teeth.

4. Three pairs of salivary glands, the parotid , sublingual , and the submandibular produce saliva that lubricates the mouth during speech and chewing and moistens food so it can be swallowed easily. Saliva also contains an enzyme called salivary amylase which begins the chemical breakdown of carbohydrates or starches . After the food is chewed and mixed with saliva, it is called a bolus .

5. What is the wavelike involuntary movement of muscles that causes the food to move in a forward direction through the digestive tract?
   —Peristalsis

6. List four (4) things that happen in the stomach during digestion.
   1) The rugae disappear
   2) cardiac sphincter closes
   3) The pyloric sphincter holds food until ready to enter the small intestine
   4) Food is converted into chyme

7. What do the following digestive juices or enzymes do to food while it is in the small intestine?
   a. maltase: } break down sugars into simpler forms
   b. sucrase:
   c. peptidases: complete the digestion of proteins
   d. bile: physically breaks down fats
   e. pancreatic amylase or amylopsin: act on sugars
   f. trypsin: act on proteins
   g. lipase or steapsin: aids the digestion of fat

8. Fingerlike projections in the small intestine, called ___villi___, contain ___blood capillaries___ and ___lacteals___. The blood capillaries absorb most of the ___digested nutrients___, while the lacteals absorb most of the digested ___fats___.

9. List three (3) functions of the large intestine.
   1) absorption of water + any remaining nutrients
   2) storage of indigestible materials before they are eliminated from the body
   3) synthesis + absorption of some B-complex vitamin

10. Name the four (4) divisions of the colon.
    1) ascending colon   3) descending colon
    2) transverse colon   4) sigmoid colon

11. List five (5) functions of the liver.
    1) produces bile to digest fats   4) produces heprin
    2) removes absorbed poisons
    3) stores vitamins, sugars, + protiens 5) produces antibodies

12. What is the function of the gallbladder?
    It stores bile + releases it into the intestine to help digest fats.

13. What is the glandular organ behind the stomach?
    The pancreas

    What two (2) secretions does it produce?
    - pancreatic juices
    - insulin

14. Name the following diseases of the digestive system.
    a. inflammation of the liver usually caused by a virus: hepatitis
    b. condition characterized by frequent watery stools: diarrhea
    c. presence of stones in the gallbladder: cholelithiasis
    d. chronic disease of the liver in which scar tissue replaces liver cells: cirrhosis
    e. dilated or varicose veins in the rectal or anal area: hemorrhoids
    f. inflammatory disease of the colon with formation of ulcers and abscesses: ulcerative colitis
    g. inflammation of mucous membrane of stomach and intestines: gastroenteritis
    h. stomach protrudes through the diaphragm by opening for esophagus: hernia

CHAPTER 6:12 URINARY SYSTEM

ASSIGNMENT SHEET

Grade _____ Name _____

INTRODUCTION: The urinary system is responsible for removing certain wastes and excess water from the body. This assignment will help you review the main facts about this system.

INSTRUCTIONS: Read the information on the Urinary System. In the space provided, print the word(s) that best completes the statement or answers the question.

1. Label the diagram of the urinary system.

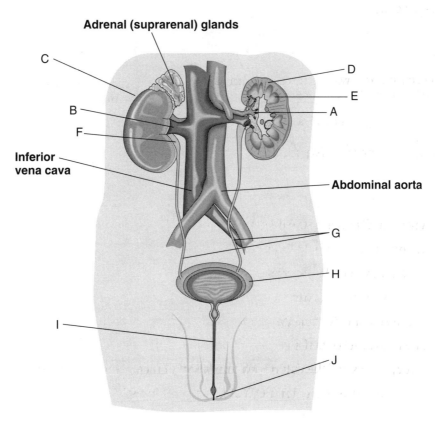

A. left renal artery

B. ~~right renal artery~~ renal vein

C. renal capsule

D. renal cortex

E. renal medulla

F. renal pelvis

G. right/left ureters

H. urinary bladder

I. urethra

J. ~~external urethral orifice~~ urinary meatus

2. Microscopic filtering units in the kidney are called _nephrons_ . The _renal_ artery carries blood to the kidney and branches of this artery carry this blood to the first part of the nephron, the _glomerulus._ As blood passes through this cluster of capillaries, _water_ , _mineral salts_ _sugar_ , _metabolic products_ and other substances are filtered out of the blood. The substances filtered out enter the next section of the nephron, _Bowman's capsule_, which passes the substances into the _convoluted tubule._ As these substances pass through various sections of the tubule, substances needed by the body are _reabsorbed_ and returned to blood _capillaries_ . Excess products such as _sugar_ and _mineral salts_, some _water_ , and _wastes_ remain in the tubule and become known as the concentrated waste liquid called _urine_ .

3. What is the rhythmic wavelike motion of the involuntary muscle of the ureter called? What does it do?
   - Peristalsis
   - moves the urine through the ureter from the kidney to the bladder

4. What are rugae? What is their function?
   - The mucous membrane lining in the bladder arranged in folds
   - they disappear to allow for expansion when the bladder fills with urine

5. How is the urethra different in males and females?
   Females
   - 1½ inches
   - opens in front of vagina
   - carries only urine to the outside

   Males
   - 8 inches
   - passes through prostate gland & out through penis
   - carries urine & semen

6. List five (5) waste products found in urine.
   1) urea   4) mineral salts
   2) uric acid   5) various pigments
   3) creatinine

7. Define the following terms.
   a. polyuria: excessive urination
   b. oliguria: below normal amounts of urination
   c. anuria: absence of urination
   d. hematuria: blood in the urine
   e. pyuria: pus in the urine
   f. nocturia: urination at night
   g. dysuria: painful urination
   h. retention: inability to empty the bladder
   i. incontinence: involuntary urination

8. An inflammation of the kidney and renal pelvis is called _pyelonephritis_ . An inflammation of the bladder is _cystitis_ . The formation of stones is _renal calculus_ . An accumulation of urinary wastes in the blood caused by kidney failure is _uremia_ .

9. What is hemodialysis?
   Removal of waste products from the blood by a hemodialysis machine.

10. Identify two (2) urinary diseases that might require a kidney transplant.
    - Renal failure
    - Uremia

CHAPTER 6:13 ENDOCRINE SYSTEM

ASSIGNMENT SHEET

Grade _____ Name _____

INTRODUCTION: The endocrine system is composed of a group of glands that secrete substances that control many body activities. This assignment will help you review the main facts about this system.

INSTRUCTIONS: Read the information on the Endocrine System. In the space provided, print the word(s) that best completes the statement or answers the question.

1. What are hormones?
   - produced & secreted by the endocrine glands
   - "chemical messangers"

   How are they transported through the body?
   - By the bloodstream

2. List five (5) functions of hormones.
   1) stimulating exocrine glands to produce secretions
   2) stimulating other endocrine glands
   3) regulating growth and developement
   4) regulating metabolism
   5) maintaing fluid & chemical balance
   6) controlling various sex processes

3. Name the endocrine glands located in the following areas of the body.
   a. above each kidney: adrenal glands
   b. on each side of the uterus in the female: ovaries
   c. under the brain in the sella turcica: pituitary gland
   d. in front of the upper part of the trachea: thyroid gland
   e. in the scrotal sac of the male: testes
   f. behind and attached to the thyroid: parathyroid gland
   g. glandular organ behind the stomach: pancreas

4. Name the hormone that performs the following function.
   a. used in metabolism of glucose: ~~adrenal Glucocorticoids~~ insulin
   b. stimulates secretion of milk: lactogenic/prolactin
   c. growth hormone, stimulates normal body growth: somatotropin
   d. regulates amount of calcium in the blood: parathormone
   e. stimulates growth and development of sex organs in male: ~~androgens follicle stimulating~~ testosterone
   f. increases metabolic rate, stimulates physical and mental growth: thyroxine & triiodothyronine
   g. stimulates growth and secretion of the thyroid gland: thyrotropin

h. activates the sympathetic nervous system: _epinephrine_

i. antidiuretic, promotes reabsorption of water in kidneys: _vassopresin_

j. regulates reabsorption of sodium in kidney and elimination of potassium: _mineralcorticoids_

k. promotes growth and development of sex organs in female: ~~follicle stimulating~~ _estrogen_

l. maintains lining of uterus: _progesterone_

5. Various diseases are listed below. Place the letter of the endocrine gland in Column B that is affected by each disease in the space provided by the disease in Column A.

Column A		Column B
1. _B_ Diabetes mellitus		A. Adrenal
2. _A_ Cushing's syndrome		B. Pancreas
3. _D_ Giantism		C. Parathyroid
4. _E_ Hyperthyroidism		D. Pituitary
5. _A_ Addison's disease		E. Thyroid
6. _D_ Acromegaly		
7. _C_ Hypoparathyroidism		
8. _E_ Cretinism		
9. _D_ Dwarfism		
10. _E_ Goiter		

6. What is the thymus? What is its function?
   - a mass of tissue located in the upper part of the chest under the sternum
   - produces thymosin

7. What is the name of the temporary endocrine gland produced during pregnancy? What happens to it after the birth of the child?
   - placenta
   - expelled after the birth of the child

8. What is the pineal body? What is its function?
   - small structure attached to the roof of the third ventricle in the brain
   - secretes 3 hormones

9. What are the gonads or sex glands of the male?
   - testes

   What are the gonads of the female?
   - ovaries

10. List six (6) symptoms of diabetes mellitus.
    - high blood sugar (hyperglycemia)
    - excessive urination (polyuria)
    - thirst (polydipsia)
    - hunger (polyphagia)
    - sugar in urine (glycosuria)
    - weight loss
    - fatigue

CHAPTER 6:14 REPRODUCTIVE SYSTEM

ASSIGNMENT SHEET

Grade _____ Name _____

INTRODUCTION: The reproductive system is responsible for the creation of new life. This assignment will help you review the main facts about this system.

INSTRUCTIONS: Read the information on the Reproductive System. In the space provided, print the word(s) that best completes the statement or answers the question.

1. Label the parts of the male reproductive system. Briefly state the function of each part.

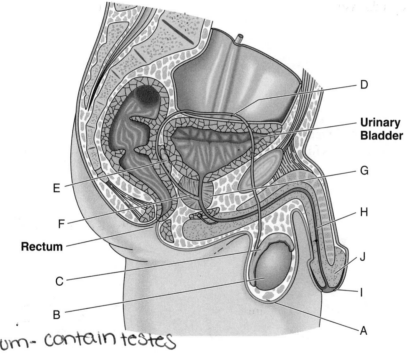

A. Scrotum - contain testes

B. Testis - produce sperm

C. Epididymis - stores sperm

D. Vas deferens - recieve sperm

E. Seminal vesicle - produce fluid to nourish sperm

F. Ejaculatory duct - carry sperm to urethra (+ semen)

G. Prostate gland - produces alkaline secretion

H. ~~Vas deferens~~ urethra - carries urine + semen

I. prepuce . foreskin

J. penis - external male reproductive organ

2. Why are the testes suspended outside the body in the scrotal sac?

The lower temperature is essential for sperm production.

3. List four (4) organs that produce a secretion that becomes a part of the semen.

1) prostate gland   3) epididymis

2) Cowpers gland   4) seminal vessicle

4. Which tube is cut to produce sterility in the male?

The vas deffens

5. A surgical removal of the prepuce is called a/an Circumcision .

6. Why is testicular self-examination important for all males? How frequently should it be done?

- To detect testicular cancer
- monthly (15 years)

7. Label the parts of the female reproductive system. Briefly state the function of each part.

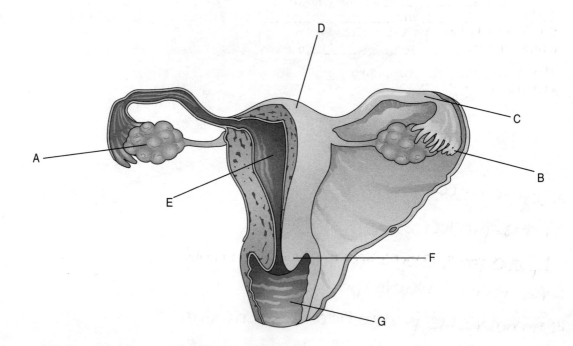

A. Ovary - contains ovum

B. Fimbriae of fallopian tube (oviduct) fingerlike - help move the ovum

C. Fallopian tube (oviduct) - passageway for the ovum to uterus

D. Fundus of uterus - top section of uterus where tubes attached

E. Uterine Cavity - Stores blood, organ of menstration, allows for baby growth + birth

F. Cervix - narrow, bottom Section that attaches to vagina

G. Vagina - connects Cervix to the uterus outside the body

8. What is fertilization? Where does it take place?

- the union of the ovum and the sperm

- fallopian tube

9. What two (2) factors keep the ovum moving through the fallopian tube toward the uterus?

~~Fimbrae of the fallopian tube~~   - peristalsis

- Cilia

10. What is the inner layer of the uterus called?

- Endometrium

What happens to this layer if fertilization does not occur?

- deteriorates & causes bleeding (menstration)

11. The structures that form the external female genital area are the ___VUlVa___.
The ___labia majora___ are two folds of fatty tissue covered with hair that
___enclose___ and ___protect___ the vagina. Two smaller folds of
tissue located within the labia majora are the ___labia minora___. An area of erectile
tissue called the ___Clitoris___ is located at the junction of the labia minora.

12. Why is it important for women to perform breast self-examinations (BSEs)? How frequently and when should a woman do a BSE?

- to detect breast cancer

- every month at the end of menstration

13. List four (4) ways to prevent contracting the human immunodeficiency virus (HIV) that causes acquired immune deficiency syndrome (AIDS).

1) Standard precautions when handling blood, body & sexual secretions

2) high risk sexual activities should be avoided

3) use a condom + spermicide

4) avoid sharing intravenous needles

14. Use the names of diseases of the reproductive systems to complete the crossword puzzle.

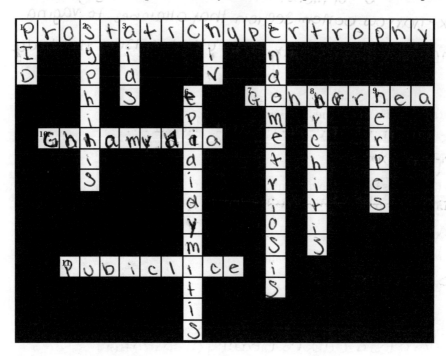

ACROSS

1. Enlargement of the prostate gland
7. STD that produces a greenish-yellow discharge in males
10. STD caused by a bacterium that lives as an intracellular parasite *Chlamydia*
11. Parasites that are transmitted sexually

DOWN

1. Abbreviation for inflammation of the cervix, endometrium, fallopian tubes, and, at times, ovaries
2. STD caused by a spirochete bacterium
3. Abbreviation for acquired immune deficiency syndrome
4. Abbreviation for the virus that causes AIDS
5. Growth of endometrial tissue outside the uterus
6. Inflammation of the epididymis
8. Inflammation of the testes
9. STD caused by a virus and characterized by fluid-filled vesicles and ulcers

CHAPTER 7:1 LIFE STAGES

ASSIGNMENT SHEET

Grade _____ Name _____

INTRODUCTION: An understanding of life stages allows a health care worker to meet individual needs and provide quality health care. This assignment will help you gain this understanding.

INSTRUCTIONS: Read the information on Life Stages. In the space provided, print the word(s) that best completes the statement or answers the question.

1. Briefly describe the four main types of growth and development that occur during each of the life stages.

   a. physical:

   b. mental:

   c. emotional:

   d. social:

2. Name the following reflex actions that allow an infant to respond to the environment.

   a. response to a loud noise or sudden movement:

   b. response to a slight touch on the cheek:

   c. response to a slight touch on the lips:

   d. response when an object is placed in the hand:

3. The following developments occur during an infant's first year of life. Put the approximate age at which they occur by the event.

   a. roll from side to back:

   b. sit unsupported for several minutes:

   c. walk without assistance:

   d. understand some words and make basic sounds:

   e. show distress, delight, anger, disgust, and fear:

   f. become shy and withdraw from strangers:

   g. mimic and imitate gestures and facial expressions:

4. The following changes occur during early childhood. List the approximate ages at which they occur.

   a. learn bladder and bowel control:

   b. make decisions based on logic instead of trial and error:

   c. make decisions based on past and present experiences:

   d. display frequent temper tantrums:

   e. show less anxiety when faced with new experiences:

   f. friends of their own age become important:

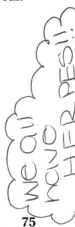

5. When a 2-year-old is admitted to a hospital, why is it important to encourage the parent(s) to bring a familiar object, such as a blanket or favorite toy, with the child?

6. Identify four (4) abstract concepts that children begin to understand in late childhood.

7. What is puberty?

8. List at least three (3) causes of conflict during the emotional development of adolescents.

9. Identify the following eating disorders.
    a. person drastically reduces food intake or refuses to eat:
    b. person alternately eats excessively or refuses to eat:
    c. person uses laxatives or induces vomiting:

10. Identify at least four (4) reasons why people use chemicals or become involved in chemical abuse.

11. A friend says, "I'd rather be dead!" Should you ignore him/her? Why or why not?

12. List at least five (5) major changes or decisions that individuals must make during early adulthood.

13. During middle adulthood, an individual can experience satisfaction or stress. List at least (3) factors that could provide satisfaction and three (3) factors that could produce stress.

<u>Satisfaction</u>   <u>Stress</u>

14. List eight (8) physical changes that might occur during late adulthood.

15. Do all individuals show physical changes of aging in their 60s and 70s?
    Why or why not?

16. List four (4) events that require emotional adjustment during late adulthood.

77

CHAPTER 7:2 DEATH AND DYING

ASSIGNMENT SHEET

Grade _____ Name _____

INTRODUCTION: Death is a part of life, and health care workers must deal with death and dying patients. This assignment will help provide some understanding about death.

INSTRUCTIONS: Read the information on Death and Dying. In the space provided, print the word(s) that best answers the question or completes the statement.

1. What is a terminal illness?

2. Identify three (3) fears that a person with a terminal illness might have.

3. Most medical personnel now feel that a patient _____ be told of his/her approaching death. However, the patient should be left with _____ and the knowledge that he/she will _____.

4. Identify the stage of dying a person is experiencing with the following statements or behaviors. Place the letter or letters of the stage from Column B in the space provided in Column A.

   Column A

   1. _____ "No, not me."

   2. _____ Promises made to God

   3. _____ Hostile and bitter

   4. _____ At peace and ready for death

   5. _____ Experiencing sadness and despair

   6. _____ "I don't believe the doctor."

   7. _____ Needs support and the presence of others

   8. _____ "Just let me live until my grandchild is born."

   9. _____ Withdraw from others

   10. _____ Refuses to discuss illness

   11. _____ Crying frequently

   12. _____ "If my husband would help more, I wouldn't be sick."

   Column B

   A. Acceptance

   B. Anger

   C. Bargaining

   D. Denial

   E. Depression

5. Do all dying patients progress through the five stages of grieving? Why or why not?

6. Before health care workers can provide care to dying patients, they must first understand their own _____ about death and come to _____ with these feelings.

7. What is the philosophy behind hospice care?

8. List three (3) types of care provided by hospice.

9. What legal documents allow a dying patient to instruct the doctor to withhold treatments that might prolong life?

10. Do you believe in the "right to die"? Why or why not?

CHAPTER 7:3 HUMAN NEEDS

ASSIGNMENT SHEET

Grade _____ Name _____

INTRODUCTION: It is important for health care workers to be aware of both their own needs and the needs of patients. This assignment will help provide an understanding of basic human needs.

INSTRUCTIONS: Read the information on Human Needs. In the space provided, print the word(s) that completes the statement or answers the question.

1. Explain what is meant by a hierarchy of needs.

2. List six (6) physiological needs.

3. Identify three (3) events that might threaten an individual's safety.

4. Why might a person hesitate to take a job with prestige and a high salary in a hospital located in an area with a high crime rate?

5. Individuals who feel safe and secure are more willing to _____ to change and more willing to face _____.

6. Identify three (3) ways in which the need for love and affection is satisfied.

7. Define *sexuality.*

8. What policy of long-term care facilities recognizes the fact that sexuality needs do not cease in late adulthood?

9. When does an individual begin to feel esteem and gain self-respect?

10. What is meant by self-actualization?

11. When needs are felt, individuals are _____ to act. If the need is met, _____ occurs. If the need is not met, _____ occurs.

12. A student, currently in the 10th grade, wants to become a respiratory therapist. The student wants to attend a private school that is very expensive. However, money is limited and the tuition is too high for her parents. List the four (4) direct methods of meeting needs and explain how this student could work to become a respiratory therapist by each method.

13. Is the use of defense mechanisms healthy or unhealthy? Why?

14. Create a situation that shows the use of each of the following defense mechanisms.

    a. rationalization:

    b. projection:

    c. displacement:

    d. compensation:

    e. daydreaming:

    f. repression:

    g. suppression:

    h. denial:

    i. withdrawal:

Name _____

15. You work in a medical laboratory. Mr. Brown is scheduled for a Glucose Tolerance Test that takes three hours to complete and requires that the patient not eat or drink anything after 12 midnight. When Mr. Brown arrives at 9:00 AM for the test, he seems angry and says, "I can't believe this stupid test is going to take three hours. Why does it take so long?"

a. Why do you think Mr. Brown is angry?

b. What would you do in this situation?

ASSIGNMENT SHEET

Grade _____   Name _____

INTRODUCTION: Communicating effectively with others is an important part of any health care. This assignment will help you review the main facts on effective communications.

INSTRUCTIONS: Read the information on Effective Communications. In the space provided, print the word(s) that completes the statement or answers the question.

1. Communication is the exchange of _____, _____, _____, and _____.

2. List four (4) factors that must be met to avoid interfering with the communication process.

3. What is wrong with the following communication processes as they relate to patients?

   a. "I think your problem is cholelithiasis."

   b. Speaking in a very soft, muted tone

   c. Radio playing loudly while preoperative care is discussed

   d. "I don't got any appointments at that time."

   e. "I don't know. Who cares?"

   f. Interrupting before the patient has finished speaking

4. Define *listening*.

5. Why does reflecting statements back to the speaker help in the communication process?

6. Nonverbal communication involves the use of _____, _____, _____, _____, and _____ to convey messages or ideas.

7. Why is it important to observe a person's nonverbal behavior?

8. Identify three (3) nonverbal ways a person can convey interest and caring.

9. List three (3) common causes of communication barriers.

10. Identify four (4) ways to improve communications with a person who is blind or visually impaired.

11. What is a common cause of anger or a negative attitude?

   List four (4) ways you can deal with an angry patient.

12. What is culture?

13. How can you deal with or react to the following situations?

   a. You are preparing a patient for surgery and all jewelry must be removed. A patient refuses to remove a religious neck chain.

   b. A patient tells you, "I don't believe in God."

   c. A patient constantly avoids eye contact while you are talking to her.

d. A patient with limited English nods his head but still seems confused as you explain a procedure.

14. Identify three (3) main barriers created by cultural diversity.

15. List four (4) senses a health care worker can use to make observations.

16. Differentiate between subjective and objective observations.

17. How should an error on a health care record be corrected?

18. Identify four (4) benefits patients experience when health care workers have effective communication skills.

CHAPTER 8 NUTRITION AND DIETS

ASSIGNMENT SHEET

Grade _____   Name _____

INTRODUCTION: A solid understanding of basic nutrition is essential for a health care worker. This assignment will help you review the main facts about proper nutrition and its relationship to good health.

INSTRUCTIONS: Read the information on Nutrition and Diets. Then follow the directions by each section to complete this assignment.

A. Matching: Place the letter of the correct word in Column B in the space provided by the definitions in Column A.

Column A	**Column B**
_____ 1. state or condition of one's nutrition	A. absorption
_____ 2. high blood pressure	B anorexia
_____ 3. state of poor nutrition caused by diet or illness	C. atherosclerosis
_____ 4. commonly called starches or sugars, major source of energy	D. carbohydrates
_____ 5. fatty substance found in body cells and animal fats	E. cholesterol
_____ 6. essential nutrients that build and repair tissue and provide heat or energy	F. digestion
_____ 7. process of breaking down food into smaller parts and changing it chemically	G. fats
_____ 8. process where blood capillaries pick up digested nutrients	H. hypertension
_____ 9. loss of appetite	I. hypotension
_____ 10. modifications of normal diet used to improve specific health conditions	J. malnutrition
	K. metabolism
	L. minerals
	M. nutritional status
	N. proteins
	O. regular diet
	P. therapeutic diet

B. Completion and Short Answer: In the space provided, print the word(s) that best completes the statement or answers the question.

1. List at least four (4) immediate effects of good nutrition.

2. A condition in which bones become porous and break easily is called _____.

3. The fibrous indigestible form of carbohydrate that provides bulk in the digestive tract is
_____.

4. List four (4) functions of fats.

5. What is the difference between saturated and unsaturated fats?

   a. List four (4) examples of saturated fats.

   b. List three (3) examples of polyunsaturated fats.

6. List three (3) functions of proteins.

   What is the difference between complete and incomplete proteins?

7. Vitamins that dissolve in water and are easily destroyed by cooking, air, and light are called
_____. Vitamins that dissolve in fat and are not easily destroyed by cooking, air, and light are called _____.

8. Identify the vitamin that performs the function listed.

   a. aids in wound healing:

   b. normal clotting of the blood:

   c. production of healthy red blood cells and metabolism of proteins:

   d. builds and maintains bones and teeth:

   e. healthy mouth tissues and eyes:

   f. structure and function of cells of skin and mucous membrane:

   g. protection of cell structure, especially red blood cells:

   h. production of antibodies:

9. Identify the mineral(s) that performs the function listed.

   a. formation of hemoglobin in red blood cells:

   b. regular heart rhythm:

   c. clotting of the blood:

   d. formation of hormones in thyroid gland:

   e. develop and maintain bones and teeth:

    f. healthy muscles and nerves:

    g. formation of hydrochloric acid:

    h. component of enzymes and insulin:

10. Identify four (4) functions of water.

     How many glasses of water should the average person drink per day?

11. What is the difference between digestion and absorption?

12. The unit of measurement used to measure the amount of heat produced during metabolism is a/an _____.

13. List four (4) factors that cause calorie requirements to vary from person to person.

14. An individual who wants to lose weight should increase _____ and decrease _____.

15. Calculate the number of calories your body requires daily to maintain your current weight. To do this, multiply your current weight in pounds by 15 calories.

     To lose one pound a week, you should decrease calorie intake by _____ calories per day. How many calories should you eat per day to lose one pound a week? _____

     To gain one pound a week, you should increase calorie intake by _____ calories per day. How many calories should you eat per day to gain one pound a week? _____

C. **Menu Plans:** Using the Food Guide Pyramid and five major food groups as a guide, create a day's menus that would fulfill the nutritional requirements of an adolescent.

<u>Breakfast</u>   <u>Lunch</u>   <u>Dinner</u>

<u>Snacks:</u> Include at least three (3).

D. Therapeutic Diets: List at least four (4) foods to limit or avoid in each of the following therapeutic diets.

<u>Diet</u>   <u>Foods to Limit or Avoid</u>

1. Soft

2. Diabetic

3. Low-calorie

4. High-calorie

5. Low-cholesterol

6. Fat-restricted

7. Sodium-restricted

8. Low-protein

9. Bland

10. Low-residue

CHAPTER 9 CULTURAL DIVERSITY

ASSIGNMENT SHEET

Grade _____ Name _____

INTRODUCTION: Every health care provider must be aware of the factors that cause each individual to be unique. This assignment will help you learn these factors.

INSTRUCTIONS: Read the information on Cultural Diversity. In the space provided, print the word(s) that best completes the statement or answers the question.

1. Define *culture.*

   Culture is the values, beliefs, attitudes, languages, symbols, rituals, behaviors, and customs unique to a particular group of people and passed from generation to generation.

2. List the four (4) basic characteristics of culture.

   1) Culture is learned
   2) Culture is shared
   3) Culture is in social nature
   4) Culture is dynamic and constantly changing

3. A classification of people based on national origin and/or culture is *Ethnicity* .
   A classification of people based on physical or biological characteristics is *Race* .
   The differences among people resulting from cultural, ethnic, and racial factors is *Cultural diversity* .

4. Do you think the United States is a "multicultural" society? Why or why not?
   Yes, there are many different cultures, races, and religions here.

5. Label each of the following statements as a bias, prejudice, or stereotype.

   a. All fat people are lazy. *Stereotype*

   b. Chemotherapy is much better than radiation to treat cancer. *Bias*

c. Herbal remedies are a waste of money. **Predjudice**

d. All teenagers are reckless drivers. **Stereotype**

e. He must be really stupid because he does not know how to use the Internet.
   Predjudice

f. Baptists are better Christians than Lutherans. **Bias**

6. Identify six (6) ways to avoid bias, prejudice, and stereotyping.

   1) know & be aware of your own values & beliefs
   2) Obtain as much info about other ethnic/cultural grou
   3) Be sensitive to behaviors & practices other than yours
   4) Develop friendships with other ethnic/cultural people
   5) Be open to differences
   6) Avoid jokes that may offend

7. What is holistic care?

   Care that provides for the well-being of the whole person (mentally, physically, emotionally)

8. Identify five (5) areas of cultural diversity.

   1) language
   2) ethics
   3) religion
   4) Beliefs
   5) gestures

9. Identify the following types of family organization.

   a. father is the authority figure: **Patriarchal**

   b. family consists of mother, father, and two children: **nuclear**

   c. parents, children, and grandparents all live in one home: **extended**

   d. mother is the authority figure: **matriarchal**

10. Identify the culture(s) that may have the following health care beliefs.

   a. illness is caused by an imbalance between yin and yang: **Asian**

   b. wearing an Azabache will treat disease: **Hispanic**

   c. health is harmony between man and nature: **South African**

   d. health is a balance between "hot and cold" forces: **Asian**

   e. evil spirits or evil "eye" cause illness: **Middle Eastern**

   f. lack of cleanliness causes illness: **European**

   g. pain must be accepted and endured silently: **Asian**

   h. tolerating pain is a sign of strength: **South African**

   i. males make decisions on the health care of the family: **Middle Eastern**

   j. shaman or medicine man is the traditional healer: **Asian**

   k. health can be maintained by diet, rest, and exercise: **European**

11. Are spirituality and religion the same? Why or why not?

   Spirituality - beliefs individuals have about themselves, their connections w/ others, + their relationship w/ a higher power

   Religion - an organized system of belief in a superhuman power or higher power

12. Why is it important for a health care provider to be aware of the beliefs about death in different religions?

To provide total care.

13. Name two (2) religions that may prohibit blood transfusions.

1) Christian Scientist

2) Jehova's Witness

14. A person who does not believe in any deity is a/an ~~through~~ Athiest . A person who believes the existence of God cannot be proved or disproved is a/an agnostic .

15. List eight (8) ways to respect cultural diversity by appreciating and respecting the personal characteristics of others.

1) Listen to patients as they express their beliefs

2) Appreciate differences in people

3) Learn more about different groups

4) Avoid bias, predjudicing, + stereotyping

5) Ask questions to determine beliefs

6) Evaluate all info before forming an opinion

7) Allow patients to practice + express beliefs

8) Respect spirituality, beliefs, religion, symbols, + practices.

16. How would you respond to the following situations?

   a. You work as a dental assistant and attempt to explain preoperative instructions to a patient who is scheduled for oral surgery. He has limited English-speaking abilities and is nodding his head yes, but he does not seem to understand the instructions.

   Find an interpreter.

   b. You work as a medical assistant and prepare a patient for a gynecological exam. She insists her husband must be in the room and states she will not undress until her husband is present.

   Allow her husband to enter.

   c. You work as a surgical technician and prepare a patient for surgery. When you tell her she must remove all jewelry, she says she never removes her cross necklace.

   Find a way that she will be able to keep it on or hold it.

   d. You work as an electrocardiograph technician and a patient has given you permission to perform an electrocardiogram. As you start to position the electrodes for each of the leads, the patient becomes very tense, pulls his arm away, and appears anxious and very nervous.

   Comfort the patient, reassure them, and explain what you're going to do.

   e. You have just started working as a geriatric assistant. As you prepare to bathe a patient, she tells you that she will wait until her daughter arrives and that her daughter will help her with her bath.

   Explain the procedure and allow the daughter to be present.

CHAPTER 10:1 MYTHS ON AGING

ASSIGNMENT SHEET

Grade _____ Name _____

INTRODUCTION: There are many myths about aging and elderly individuals. This assignment will help you distinguish between myths and facts.

INSTRUCTIONS: Read the information on Myths on Aging. Then read the statements below. If the statement is a fact, put a check in the "Fact" column. If the statement is a myth, put a check in the "Myth" column. Then write why the statement is a myth in the space provided.

<u>Fact</u>   <u>Myth</u>

_____   _____   1. Aging is a normal process that leads to normal changes in body structure and function.

_____   _____   2. Most elderly individuals experience confusion and disorientation.

_____   _____   3. Over 2 million people will be cared for in long-term care facilities by the year 2008.

_____   _____   4. Many individuals are active, productive, and self-sufficient into their 80s and 90s.

_____   _____   5. The majority of the elderly live in poverty.

_____   _____   6. Older people are usually lonely and unhappy.

_____   _____   7. Most individuals lose interest in work at age 60 and make plans to retire.

_____   _____   8. Old age begins at age 65.

_____   _____   9. Most elderly individuals live in their own home or apartment or with other family members.

_____   _____   10. Retired people are usually bored and have nothing to do with their lives.

CHAPTER 10:2 PHYSICAL CHANGES OF AGING

ASSIGNMENT SHEET

Grade _____ Name _____

INTRODUCTION: Physical changes are a normal part of the aging process. This assignment will help you learn the main physical changes.

INSTRUCTIONS: Read the information on Physical Changes of Aging. In the space provided, print the word(s) that best completes the statement or answers the question.

1. Most physical changes that occur with aging are _____ and take place over a/an _____ of time. In addition, the _____ and _____ of change varies with different individuals. Previous _____, _____, _____ status, and _____ environment can also have an effect. If an individual can recognize the changes as a/an _____ part of aging, the individual can usually learn to _____ and _____ with the changes.

2. List three (3) physical changes that may occur in each of the following systems.

   a. integumentary:

   b. musculoskeletal:

   c. circulatory:

   d. respiratory:

   e. nervous:

   f. digestive:

   g. urinary:

   h. endocrine:

   i. reproductive:

3. Identify the following common diseases or conditions in the elderly.

   a. calcium and minerals are lost from bones and bones become brittle and more likely to fracture:

   b. inflammation of the joints:

   c. formation of a blood clot:

   d. alveoli lose their elasticity:

   e. lens of eye becomes cloudy or opaque:

   f. increased intraocular pressure in the eye:

   g. difficulty in swallowing:

h. inability to control urination:

i. dark yellow or brown colored spots on the skin:

4. In each of the following situations, a physical change of aging has occurred. Briefly describe how a health care worker can assist the individual in learning how to cope or adapt to the change.

a. Mrs. Darbey complains of dry and itchy skin.

b. Mr. Polinski constantly complains of feeling cold.

c. Mr. Stark is irritable and tired during the day because he gets up three or four times at night to urinate.

d. Because of arthritis, Mrs. Mendosa is unable to button her blouses. However, she insists on dressing herself.

e. Mr. Pease lives at home but refuses to take a bath. He is afraid of falling in the tub.

f. Mrs. Webber refuses to sleep in a bed because she becomes short of breath while lying down.

g. Mr. Chang uses excessive salt, pepper, and sugar on all his food but still complains that the food has no taste.

h. Mrs. Pearce wants to exercise and walk two miles each day, but she gets very tired and short of breath.

i. Mr. Mende constantly talks very loudly and asks everyone to speak up or repeat what has been said.

j. Mrs. Valentino refuses to leave her room because she says, "I have been wetting my pants, and it is embarrassing."

CHAPTER 10:3 PSYCHOSOCIAL CHANGES OF AGING

ASSIGNMENT SHEET

Grade _____ Name _____

INTRODUCTION: Elderly individuals experience psychological and social changes along with physical changes. This assignment will help provide an understanding of these changes.

INSTRUCTIONS: Read the information on Psychosocial Changes in Aging. In the space provided, print the word(s) that best completes the statement or answers the question.

1. Some individuals cope with psychosocial changes, and others experience extreme _____ and _____.

2. List two (2) things a person might do after retirement to find a satisfactory replacement for the role their job played.

3. List three (3) causes for the sense of loss some individuals feel at retirement.

4. Identify two (2) factors that can cause a change in social relationships for an elderly individual.

5. Identify two (2) ways an individual can adjust to social changes when a spouse and friends die.

6. Why does a move to a long-term care facility usually create stress in elderly individuals?

7. Identify two (2) ways an individual can be given the opportunity to create a "home" environment in a long-term care facility.

8. List three (3) factors that can lead to a loss of independence in the elderly.

9. How can a health care worker allow an elderly individual as much independence as possible?

10. How does a disease differ from a disability?

11. Identify four (4) fears experienced by a sick person.

12. Identify two (2) ways a health care worker can help an individual deal with the fears created by an illness.

CHAPTER 10:4 CONFUSION AND DISORIENTATION IN THE ELDERLY

ASSIGNMENT SHEET

Grade _____ Name _____

INTRODUCTION: This assignment will help you gain an understanding of how to care for a confused or disorientated individual.

INSTRUCTIONS: Read the information on Confusion and Disorientation in the Elderly. In the space provided, print the word(s) that best completes the statement or answers the question.

1. List six (6) signs of confusion or disorientation.

2. Name six (6) causes of temporary confusion or disorientation.

3. Name the following diseases that can cause chronic confusion or disorientation.

   a. blood clot obstructs blood flow to brain:

   b. walls of blood vessels become thick and lose elasticity:

   c. walls of blood vessels become narrow from deposits of fat and minerals:

4. How does acute dementia differ from chronic dementia?

5. Each of the following changes can occur in a patient with Alzheimer's disease. Identify the stage at which the change occurs by putting "early," "middle," or "terminal" by each symptom.

   a. paranoia and hallucinations increase:

   b. incoherent and not able to communicate with words:

   c. total disorientation regarding person, time, and place:

   d. inability to plan and follow through with activities of daily living:

   e. restlessness at night:

f. loses control of bladder and bowel function:

g. mood and personality changes:

h. personal hygiene ignored:

i. perseveration or repetitious behavior occurs:

6. Certain aspects of care should be followed with any confused or disorientated individual. Provide a/an _____ and _____ environment, follow the same _____, keep activities _____, and avoid loud _____, _____ rooms, and excessive _____. Promote awareness of person, time, and place by providing _____.

7. How can a health care worker use reality orientation to correct or improve the following situations?

a. Mrs. Probasco is confused about time and cannot read her watch.

b. Mrs. Mendez wants to sleep all day and wander all night.

c. Many assistants call Mr. Blanton "Grandpa," and he does not know his name.

d. Mr. Pearson keeps calling you "Janet," which is his wife's name.

e. Mrs. Handwork likes to walk in the hall but cannot find her own room. She does recognize pictures of herself.

f. Mrs. Zimmerman wears a hearing aid but does not appear to hear most conversations.

8. True–False: Circle the T if the statement is true. Circle the F if the statement is false.

T   F   a. Caring for a confused or disoriented individual can be frustrating and even frightening.

T   F   b. Transient ischemic attacks (TIAs) cause a temporary period of diminished blood flow to the brain.

T   F   c. Elderly individuals are more sensitive to medications.

T   F   d. A high fever can cause chronic dementia.

T   F   e. Alzheimer's disease is caused by a genetic defect.

T   F   f. Bingo games and large group activities help a confused individual by providing mental stimulation.

T   F   g. When a disoriented patient makes an incorrect statement, agree with the patient.

T   F   h. Patience, consistency, and sincere caring are essential when dealing with confusion and disorientation.

T   F   i. In later stages of confusion and disorientation, when the individual is not able to respond, reality orientation can cause increased anxiety and agitation.

CHAPTER 10:5 MEETING THE NEEDS OF THE ELDERLY

ASSIGNMENT SHEET

Grade _____ Name _____

INTRODUCTION: This assignment will help you to identify and learn how to meet the needs of an elderly individual.

INSTRUCTIONS: Read the information on Meeting the Needs of the Elderly. In the space provided, print the word(s) that best completes the statement or answers the question.

1. Elderly individuals have the same _____ and _____needs of any person at any age. However, these needs are sometimes intensified by _____or _____ changes that disrupt the normal life pattern.

2. List six (6) areas that can be affected by an individual's culture.

3. The spiritual beliefs and practices of an individual are called their _____. It is important to accept an individual's belief without _____. Health care workers must not force their own _____ on the individuals they are caring for.

4. List three (3) ways a health care worker can show respect and consideration of a person's religious beliefs.

5. Identify four (4) types of abuse.

6. You see a fellow worker push Mr. Davis into a chair and say, "I am sick and tired of your wandering outside. You stay in this chair until I get back or I'll tie you in."

   What type(s) of abuse might this represent?

   What should you do?

7. You work as a medical assistant. A daughter, who brings her mother, Mrs. Kupin, to the office says, "She wets the bed constantly, and I can't stand it any more." Mrs. Kupin is 92 years old and lives with her daughter. As you help prepare her for an examination, you observe that she is very thin, has bruises and scratches on her arms and legs, and seems confused. Mrs. Kupin asks, "Where am I? Is this a nursing home?"

What type(s) of abuse might this represent?

What should you do?

8. Why do elderly individuals who are abused hesitate or refuse to report abuse?

9. Why are patients' rights important?

10. In its Older Americans Act, the federal government established a/an _____ Program. This is a specially trained individual who may _____ and try to _____ complaints, suggest _____ for health care, _____ and _____ state and/or federal regulations, report _____ to the correct agency, and provide _____ for individuals involved in the care of the elderly.

CHAPTER 11:1 USING BODY MECHANICS

ASSIGNMENT SHEET

Grade _____ Name _____

INTRODUCTION: The correct use of body mechanics is essential to protect both the worker and the patient. This sheet will allow you to review the main facts.

INSTRUCTIONS: Review the information in the text about Using Body Mechanics. Put the text aside and answer the following questions. Print your answers in the spaces provided.

1. Define body mechanics.

2. List three (3) reasons for using correct body mechanics.

3. In the following diagrams, certain rules for correct body mechanics are not being observed. At least three rules are being broken in each diagram. In the space provided for each diagram, list three rules not being observed.

Diagram 1:

(1)

(2)

(3)

Diagram 2:

(1)

(2)

(3)

Diagram 3:

(1)

(2)

(3)

Name _____ Date _____

Evaluated by _____

DIRECTIONS: Practice body mechanics according to the criteria listed. When you are ready for your final check, give this sheet to your instructor for evaluation.

PROFICIENT

Using Body Mechanics	Points Possible	Peer Check		Final Check*		Points Earned**	Comments
		Yes	No	Yes	No		
1. Demonstrates broad base of support:							
Keeps feet 8 to 10 inches apart	5						
Puts one foot slightly forward	5						
Points toes in direction of movement	5						
Balances weight on both feet	5						
2. Picks up heavy object:							
Gets close to object	6						
Maintains broad base of support	6						
Bends from hips and knees	6						
Uses strongest muscles	6						
3. Pushes heavy object:							
Gets close to object	8						
Maintains broad base of support	8						
Uses weight of body	8						
4. Carries heavy object:							
Keeps object close to body	8						
Uses strongest muscles	8						
5. Changes directions:							
Maintains broad base of support	8						
Turns with feet and entire body	8						
Totals	100						

* Final Check: Instructor or authorized person evaluates.
** Points Earned: Points possible times each "yes" check.

CHAPTER 11:2 PREVENTING ACCIDENTS AND INJURIES

ASSIGNMENT SHEET

Grade _____ Name _____

INTRODUCTION: Safety standards have been established to protect you and the patient. This sheet will help you to review the main standards.

INSTRUCTIONS: Read the information sheet on Preventing Accidents and Injuries. In the space provided, print the word(s) that best completes the statement or answers the question.

1. What is OSHA? What is its purpose?

2. List four (4) types of information that must be included on Material Safety Data Sheets (MSDSs).

3. What is the hazardous ingredient in Clorox bleach? (Hint: Review the MSDS figure in the textbook.)

4. Identify four (4) body fluids included in the bloodborne pathogen standard.

5. Name the three (3) main diseases that can be contracted by exposure to body fluids.

6. List four (4) rules or standards to observe while working with solutions in the laboratory.

7. List four (4) rules or standards to observe while working with equipment in the laboratory.

8. Before you perform any procedure on patients, there are several standards you must observe. List four (4) of these standards.

9. Identify two (2) ways to show respect for a patient's right to privacy.

10. What are two (2) methods you can use to correctly identify a patient?

11. List five (5) safety checkpoints that should be observed before leaving a patient or resident in a bed.

12. When should hands be washed?

13. When should safety glasses be worn?

14. Briefly state how you should handle the following situations.

    a. You cut your hand slightly on a piece of glass:

    b. You get a particle in your eye:

    c. You turn a piece of equipment on, but it does not run correctly:

    d. You spill an acid solution on the counter:

    e. You start to plug in an electrical cord and notice that the third prong for grounding has been broken off:

Name _____ Date _____

Evaluated by _____

DIRECTIONS: Practice safety according to the criteria listed. When you are ready for your final check, give this sheet to your instructor. Given simulated situations and using the proper equipment and supplies, you will be expected to respond orally or demonstrate the following safety criteria.

PROFICIENT

Preventing Accidents and Injuries	Points Possible	Peer Check Yes	No	Final Check* Yes	No	Points Earned**	Comments
1. Wears required laboratory uniform	5						
2. Walks in the laboratory area	5						
3. Reports injuries, accidents, and unsafe situations	5						
4. Keeps area clean and replaces supplies	5						
5. Washes hands frequently as needed	5						
6. Dries hands before handling electrical equipment	5						
7. Wears safety glasses	5						
8. Avoids horseplay	5						
9. Flushes solutions out of eyes or off of skin	5						
10. Informs instructor if particle gets in eye	5						
11. Operates equipment only after taught	5						
12. Reads instructions accompanying equipment	5						
13. Reports damaged or malfunctioning equipment	5						
14. Reads Material Safely Data Sheets (MSDSs) provided with hazardous chemicals	5						
15. Reads labels on solution bottles 3 times	5						
16. Handles solutions carefully to avoid contact with skin and eyes	5						
17. Reports broken equipment or spilled solutions	5						
18. Identifies patients in two (2) ways	5						
19. Explains procedures to patients	5						
20. Observes patients closely during any procedure	5						
Totals	100						

*   Final Check: Instructor or authorized person evaluates.
** Points Earned: Points possible times each "yes" check.

CHAPTER 11:3 OBSERVING FIRE SAFETY

ASSIGNMENT SHEET

Grade _____ Name _____

INTRODUCTION: Knowing how to respond to a fire can save your life. This sheet will help you review the main facts of fire safety.

INSTRUCTIONS: Read the text information about Observing Fire Safety. In the space provided, print the word(s) that best completes the statement or answers the question.

1. Fires need three (3) things to start. What are they?

2. List four (4) causes of fires.

3. List three (3) rules for preventing fires.

4. Where is the nearest fire alarm box located?

5. a. What is the location of the nearest fire extinguisher?

   b. What class of fire extinguisher is it? What kind of fire will it extinguish?

6. Fill in the following chart about fire extinguishers.

Class	Contains	Used on what type of fires?
A		
B		
C		
ABC		

7. For what does the acronym *RACE* stand?

   R:

   A:

   C:

   E:

8. List three (3) special precautions that must be observed when a patient is receiving oxygen.

9. Identify three (3) basic principles that must be followed when any type of disaster occurs.

10. Health care workers are _____ responsible for familiarizing themselves with disaster policies so appropriate action can be taken when a disaster strikes.

Name _____   Date _____

Evaluated by _____

DIRECTIONS: Practice fire safety according to the criteria listed. When you are ready for your final check, give this sheet to your instructor.

PROFICIENT

Observing Fire Safety	Points Possible	Peer Check Yes	No	Final Check* Yes	No	Points Earned**	Comments
1. Identifies nearest alarm box	9						
2. Sounds alarm correctly	9						
3. Points out locations of extinguishers in area	9						
4. Selects correct extinguisher for following types of fires:							
Burning paper	5						
Burning oil	5						
Electrical fire	5						
5. Simulates the operation of an extinguisher:							
Checks type	5						
Releases lock	5						
Holds firmly	5						
Stands 6 to 10 feet away from edge	5						
Aims at fire	5						
Discharges correctly	5						
Uses side-to-side motion	5						
Sprays at near edge at bottom of fire	5						
6. Replaces or has extinguisher recharged after use	9						
7. Evacuates laboratory or clinical area following established policy for fires	9						
Totals	100						

* Final Check: Instructor or authorized person evaluates.
** Points Earned: Points possible times each "yes" check.

CHAPTER 11 SAFETY EXAMINATION

Grade _____ Name _____

Read all directions carefully. Put your name on all pages of the examination.

Multiple Choice: In the space provided, place the letter of the answer that best completes the statement or answers the question.

_____ 1. Operate a piece of equipment only when

    a. you have been instructed on how to use it

    b. you see other students using it

    c. you think you know how to handle it

    d. you have similar equipment in other classes

_____ 2. If you find a damaged piece of equipment

    a. dispose of it immediately

    b. report it to the instructor

    c. use it but be very careful

    d. repair it yourself before you use it

_____ 3. Solutions that will be used in the laboratory

    a. can be injurious, so avoid eye and skin contact

    b. can be mixed together in most cases

    c. do not always need a label

    d. are all safe for your use

_____ 4. When the instructor is out of the room

    a. equipment should not be operated

    b. it is all right to operate equipment

    c. it is a good time to experiment with equipment

    d. be extra careful when using equipment

_____ 5. All injuries obtained in the laboratory

    a. should be treated by a fellow student

    b. can be ignored if minor

    c. should be washed with soap and water

    d. should be reported to the instructor

_____ 6. If a particle gets in your eye, you should

    a. rub your eye

    b. use cotton to remove it

    c. call the instructor

    d. flush your eye with water to remove it

_____ 7. When handling any electrical equipment, be sure to

    a. wash your hands immediately before handling it

    b. check first for damaged cords or improper grounds

    c. plug equipment carefully into any socket

    d. ask for written instructions on how to use it

_____ 8. Horseplay or practical jokes

    a. are permitted if no one is insulted

    b. may be done during breaks or study time

    c. cause accidents and have no place in the lab

    d. usually do not result in accidents

_____ 9. The major cause of fires is

    a. smoking and matches

    b. defects in heating systems

    c. improper rubbish disposal

    d. misuse of electricity

_____ 10. The three things needed to start a fire are

    a. air, oxygen, and fuel

    b. fuel, heat, and oxygen

    c. fuel, carbon dioxide, and heat

    d. air, carbon dioxide, and fuel

_____ 11. Injuries are more likely to happen to persons who

    a. take chances

    b. use equipment properly

    c. practice safety

    d. respect the dangers in using equipment

_____ 12. If your personal safety is in danger because of fire

    a. get the fire extinguisher and put it out

    b. run out of the area as fast as you can

    c. leave the area quietly and in an orderly fashion

    d. open all windows and doors

_____ 13. Wearing safety glasses in a laboratory

    a. is never necessary

    b. should be done if you think it is necessary

    c. is a requirement at all times

    d. is required for certain procedures

True–False: Circle the T if the statement is true. Circle the F if the statement is false.

T   F   14. Carbon dioxide fire extinguishers leave a residue or snow that can cause burns or eye irritations.

T   F   15. Spilled solutions, such as bleach, should be wiped up immediately.

T   F   16. Laboratory uniforms are worn for protection and as a safety measure.

T   F   17. If any solution comes in contact with your skin or eyes, flush the area with water and call the instructor.

T   F   18.   The third prong on an electric plug is important for grounding electrical equipment.

T   F   19.   In case of a fire alarm, avoid panic.

T   F   20.   Correct body mechanics should be used while performing procedures.

T   F   21.   Class A fire extinguishers can be used on electrical fires.

T   F   22.   While using a fire extinguisher, hold the extinguisher firmly and direct it to the middle or main part of the fire.

T   F   23.   Smoke and panic kill more people in fires than the fire itself.

T   F   24.   For your own safety and the safety of a patient, it is important that you wash your hands frequently.

T   F   25.   All waste material should be disposed of in the nearest available container.

T   F   26.   All solutions used in the laboratory are poisonous.

T   F   27.   You should read the bottle label of any solution that you use at least three (3) times.

T   F   28.   All manufacturers must provide a Material Safety Data Sheet (MSDS) with any hazardous product they sell.

T   F   29.   When lifting a patient in bed, a narrow base of support should be maintained.

T   F   30.   Keep the feet apart and the knees flexed when picking up an item from the floor.

31. Fill in the following chart with the indicated information.

Type Fire Extinguisher	Contains	Used on what type of fire?
a.		
b.		
c.		
d.		

32. List three (3) rules for preventing fires.

33. What is OSHA? What is its purpose?

34. How can you determine precautions that should be followed while using a hazardous chemical?

35. Identify the three (3) main diseases that can be contracted by exposure to body fluids.

ASSIGNMENT SHEET

Grade _____ Name _____

INTRODUCTION: This assignment will allow you to gain a basic knowledge of how disease is transmitted and the main ways to prevent it.

INSTRUCTIONS: Read the information on Understanding the Principles of Infection Control. In the space provided, print the word(s) that best completes the statement or answers the question.

1. Use the Key Terms to complete the crossword puzzle.

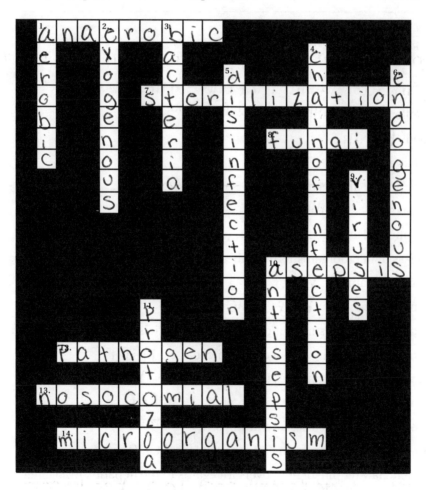

ACROSS

1. Organisms that live and reproduce in the absence of oxygen

7. Process that destroys all microorganisms including spores and viruses

8. Plantlike organisms that live on dead organic matter

10. Absence of pathogens

12. Germ- or disease-producing microorganism

13. Infections acquired in a health care facility

14. Small living plant or animal organism not visible to naked eye

DOWN

1. Organisms that require oxygen to live

2. Disease originates outside the body

3. One-celled plantlike organisms that multiply rapidly

4. Factors that must be present for disease to occur

5. Process that destroys or kills pathogens

6. Disease originates within the body

9. Smallest microorganisms

10. Process that inhibits or prevents the growth of pathogenic organisms

11. One-celled animal organisms found in decayed materials and contaminated water

---

2. How do nonpathogens differ from pathogens?

   - Nonpathogen: microorganisms that are beneficial in maintaining certain body processes
   - Pathogen: microorganisms that cause infection and disease

3. Identify the following shapes of bacteria.

   a. rod shaped: Bacilli

   b. comma shaped: Vibro (Spirilla)

   c. round or spherical arranged in a chain: Streptococci

   d. spiral or corkscrew: Spirilla

   e. round or spherical arranged in clusters: Staphylococci

4. Identify the class of microorganisms described by the following statements.

   a. smallest microorganisms: Virus

   b. parasitic microorganisms: Rickettsiae

   c. one-celled animal organisms found in decayed materials and contaminated water: Protozoa

   d. plantlike organisms that live on dead organic matter: Fungi

   e. microorganisms that live on fleas, lice, ticks, and mites: Rickettsiae

   f. cause diseases such as gonorrhea and syphilis: Bacteria

   g. cause diseases such as measles and mumps: Protozoa Virus

   h. cause diseases such as ringworm and athlete's foot: Fungi

5. What does federal law require of employers in regards to the hepatitis B vaccine?
   It must be provided w/ no cost to all healthcare workers w/ occupational exposure to blood and other bodily secretions.

6. List three (3) things needed for microorganisms to grow and reproduce.
   1) warm environment
   2) darkness
   3) moisture

7. Identify two (2) ways pathogenic organisms can cause infection and disease.
   1) Pathogens produce poision(toxins)
   2) Pathogens cause allergic reactions

8. What is the difference between an endogenous disease and an exogenous disease?
   - <u>Endogenous</u>: infection/disease originates w/i the body
   - <u>Exogenous</u>: infection/disease originates outside the body

9. Name three (3) common examples of nosocomial infections.
   1) Staphylococcus
   2) Psuedomonas
   3) Enterococci
   What do health care facilities do to prevent and deal with nosocomial infections?
   Use infection control programs.

10. Identify the part(s) of the chain of infection that has been eliminated by the following actions.
    a. thorough washing of the hands: Portal of ~~Entry~~ Exit
    b. intact unbroken skin: Portal of Entry
    c. healthy, well rested individual: Susceptible Host
    d. cleaning and sterilizing a blood covered instrument: ~~Causitive Agent~~ Source of Resivoir
    e. spraying to destroy mosquitoes: ~~Causitive Agent~~ Mode of Transmission
    f. rapid, accurate identification of organisms: Causitive Agent

11. List four (4) common aseptic techniques.
    1) Handwashing
    2) Good Personal Hygeine
    3) Use of disposable gloves
    4) Proper cleaning of instruments & equipment

12. Define the following.
    a. antisepsis: prevention + inhibition of growth of pathogenic organisms (not effective against spores/viruses)

    b. disinfection: destruction/killing of pathogenic organisms

    c. sterilization: destroys all microorganisms

CHAPTER 12:2 WASHING HANDS

ASSIGNMENT SHEET

Grade _____ Name _____

INTRODUCTION: Handwashing is the most important method used to practice aseptic technique. This assignment will help you review the main facts.

INSTRUCTIONS: Read the information on Washing Hands. In the space provided, print the word(s) that best completes the statement or answers the question.

1. What is an aseptic technique?
   A method followed to prevent the spread of germs or pathogens.

2. List two (2) reasons for washing the hands.
   1) Helps prevent + control the spread of pathogens from one person to another.
   2) Helps protect the health worker from disease and illness.

3. List six (6) times the hands should be washed.
   1) When you arrive at the facility and immediately before leaving
   2) Before/after every patient contact
   3) Any time the hands become contaminated during a procedure
   4) Before applying and immediately after removing gloves
   5) Before + after handling any specimen
   6) After contact w/ any soiled/contaminated item

4. Why is soap used as a cleansing agent?
   It aids in the removal of germs through its sudsy action and alkali content.

5. How should the fingertips be pointed while washing hands?
   Downward

   Why?
   To prevent water from getting on the forearms and running down to contaminate the clean hands.

6. What temperature water should be used?
   Warm

   Why?
   It is less damaging on the skin than hot water and creates a better lather than cold water.

7. Why are paper towels used while turning on and off the faucet?
   To prevent contamination of the hands from pathogens on the faucet.

8. List three (3) surfaces on the hands that must be cleaned.
   1) palms   2) backs + tops   3) area between fingers

9. Name two (2) items that can be used to clean the nails.
   1) cuticle stick
   2) brush

Name _____ Date _____

Evaluated by _____

DIRECTIONS: Practice washing hands according to the criteria listed. When you are ready for your final check, give this sheet to your instructor.

PROFICIENT

Washing Hands	Points Possible	Peer Check Yes	No	Final Check* Yes	No	Points Earned**	Comments
1. Assembles supplies	5						
2. Turns faucet on with dry towel	6						
3. Regulates temperature of water	6						
4. Wets hands with fingertips pointed down	7						
5. Gets soapy lather	6						
6. Scrubs palms using friction and a circular motion for 10 to 15 seconds	7						
7. Scrubs tops of hands with opposite palms	7						
8. Interlaces fingers to wash between	7						
9. Cleans nails:							
With small brush	5						
Uses blunt edge of orange stick	5						
10. Rinses with fingertips pointed down	7						
11. Dries thoroughly	7						
12. Places towels in waste can	6						
13. Turns off faucet with dry towel	7						
14. Leaves area neat and clean	5						
15. Identifies five (5) times hands must be washed	7						
Totals	100						

* Final Check: Instructor or authorized person evaluates.
** Points Earned: Points possible times each "yes" check.

CHAPTER 12:3 OBSERVING STANDARD PRECAUTIONS

ASSIGNMENT SHEET

Grade _____ Name _____

INTRODUCTION: Observing standard precautions is one way the chain of infection can be broken. This assignment will allow you to review the main principles of standard precautions.

INSTRUCTIONS: Read the information on Observing Standard Precautions. In the space provided, print the word(s) that best completes the statement or answers the question.

1. Name three (3) pathogens spread by blood and body fluids that are a major concern to health care workers.
   1) Hepatitis B
   2) Hepatitis C
   3) AIDS

2. What federal agency established standards for contamination with blood or body fluids that must be followed by all health care facilities?
   Occupational Safety and Health Administration (OSHA)

3. Name four (4) types of personal protective equipment (PPE) that an employer must provide.
   1) gloves   3) lab coat
   2) gown   4) masks

4. Can a health care worker drink coffee in a laboratory where blood tests are performed? Why or why not?
   No, it can be contaminated by bodily fluids.

5. What responsibilities does an employer have if an employee is splashed with blood when a tube containing blood breaks?
   Provide a confidential medical evaluation and follow-up.

6. List the four (4) main requirements that employers must meet as a result of the Needlestick Safety and Prevention Act.
   1) Identify and use effective and safer medical devices.
   2) Incorporate changes in annual update of Exposure Control Plan.
   3) Solicit input from nonmanagerial employees who are responsible for direct patient care.
   4) Maintain a sharps injury log.

7. When must standard precautions be used?
   At all times

8. Describe four (4) situations when gloves must be worn.

1) When in contact w/ blood, body fluids, secretions, excretions, mucous membranes, tissue specimens, or nonintact skin

2) handling/cleaning contaminated items/surfaces

3) Performing invasive procedures

4) Performing venipuncture/blood tests

9. When must gowns be worn?

During any procedure that is likely to cause splashing or spraying of blood, body fluids, secretions, or excretions.

10. Describe three (3) examples of situations when masks, protective eyewear, or face shields must be worn.

During procedures that may produce splashes or sprays of blood, body fluids, secretions, or excretions, such as irrigation of wounds, suctioning, dental procedures, delivery of a baby, and surgical procedures.

11. When must masks be changed?

- every 30 minutes
- when they become moist/wet

12. How must needles and syringes be handled after use?

They must be left uncapped and attatched to the syringe and placed in a leak proof, puncture resistant sharps container thats labled with a red biohazard symbol.

13. During a blood test, some blood splashes on the laboratory counter. How must it be removed?

While wearing gloves, wipe the area w/ disposable cleaning cloths. Then clean the area w/ a disinfectant solution. Place materials in an infectious waste container.

14. What is the purpose of mouthpieces or resuscitation devices?

To avoid mouth to mouth resuscitation.

15. Where must you discard a dressing contaminated with blood and pus?

In a special infectious waste or biohazardous material bag.

16. What must you do if you stick yourself with a contaminated needle?

It must be reported immediately and then the agency policy must be followed immediately.

Name _____ Date _____

Evaluated by _____

DIRECTIONS: Practice observing standard precautions according to the criteria listed. When you are ready for your final check, give this sheet to your instructor.

PROFICIENT

Observing Standard Precautions	Points Possible	Peer Check Yes	No	Final Check* Yes	No	Points Earned**	Comments
1. Assembles equipment and supplies	3						
2. Washes hands correctly	4						
3. Puts on gloves if:							
Contacting blood, body fluid, secretions, excretions, mucous membranes, or nonintact skin	3						
Handling contaminated items/surfaces	3						
Performing invasive procedures	3						
Performing blood tests	3						
4. Removes gloves correctly:							
Grasps outside of cuff of first glove	3						
Pulls glove down and turns inside out	3						
Places fingers inside cuff of second glove	4						
Pulls glove down and turns inside out	3						
Disposes of glove correctly	3						
Washes hands immediately	3						
5. Puts on gown if splashing of blood/body fluid likely	4						
6. Removes gown correctly:							
Handles only inside while removing	2						
Folds gown inward	2						
Rolls gown	2						
Places in proper laundry bag	2						
7. Wears masks and protective eyewear if needed:							
Puts on if droplets of blood/body fluid likely	3						
Handles only ties of mask when removing	3						
Cleans and disinfects protective eyewear	3						
8. Disposes of sharps correctly	4						

12:3 (cont.)

Observing Standard Precautions	Points Possible	Peer Check Yes	No	Final Check* Yes	No	Points Earned**	Comments
9. Wipes up spills/splashes of blood/body fluids:							
Puts on gloves	2						
Wipes up spill with disposable cloths/ gauze	2						
Discards cloths/gauze in infectious waste bag	2						
Wipes area with clean cloth/gauze and disinfectant	2						
Discards cloths/gauze in infectious waste bag	2						
Removes gloves	2						
Washes hands immediately	2						
10. Handles infectious waste bags correctly:							
Forms cuff at top before using	2						
Discards infectious waste in bag	2						
Wears gloves to close bag	2						
Puts hands under cuff	2						
Expels excess air gently	2						
Folds top edges to seal bag	2						
Tapes or ties bag	2						
11. Uses mouthpieces or resuscitation devices correctly	4						
12. Replaces equipment	3						
13. Washes hands	3						
Totals	100						

* Final Check: Instructor or authorized person evaluates.
** Points Earned: Points possible times each "yes" check.

CHAPTER 12:4 STERILIZING WITH AN AUTOCLAVE

ASSIGNMENT SHEET

Grade _____ Name _____

INTRODUCTION: In order to use an autoclave correctly, you must know the following information. Read the information on Sterilizing with an Autoclave and proceed with this assignment.

INSTRUCTIONS: In the space provided, print the answer to each question.

1. The autoclave uses _____ under _____ or _____ to sterilize equipment and supplies. It will destroy all _____, both _____ and _____, including _____ and _____.

2. What must be done to any equipment or supplies before they are sterilized in the autoclave?

3. List three (3) types of wraps that can be used in the autoclave.

4. Why are autoclave indicators used?

5. List two (2) types of autoclave indicators.

6. List three (3) rules that must be followed while loading an autoclave.

7. Why is it important to separate loads before sterilizing them in an autoclave?

8. How do you determine the correct time and temperature for sterilizing different articles in the autoclave?

9. Why do items have to be dry before being removed from an autoclave?

10. Where should sterilized items be stored?

11. How long do items remain sterile after autoclaving?

12. The wrap on a sterile bowl is wet. What should you do?

13. What is the minimum temperature required for dry heat sterilization?

    What is the minimum time required for dry heat sterilization?

14. Identify two (2) items for which dry heat sterilization is more effective.

Name _____ Date _____

Evaluated by _____

DIRECTIONS: Practice wrapping items for autoclaving according to the criteria listed. When you are ready for your final check, give this sheet to your instructor.

PROFICIENT

Wrapping Items for Autoclaving	Points Possible	Peer Check Yes	No	Final Check* Yes	No	Points Earned**	Comments
1. Assembles equipment and supplies	2						
2. Washes hands and puts on gloves	3						
3. Sanitizes item to be sterilized:							
Cleans with soapy water	2						
Rinses in cool water	2						
Rinses in hot water	2						
Dries item thoroughly	2						
Wears gloves if item contaminated with blood/body fluids	3						
Brushes serrated instruments	3						
4. Prepares linen for wrapping:							
Checks that linen is clean and dry	3						
Folds in half lengthwise	3						
Fanfolds into even sections	3						
Turns back corner tab	3						
5. Selects correct wrap for item	3						
6. Places item in center of wrap	3						
Leaves hinged instruments open	3						
7. Folds bottom corner up to center	3						
Folds back corner tab	3						
8. Folds a side corner in to center	3						
Seals edges and removes air pockets	3						
Folds back corner tab	3						
9. Folds other side corner in to center	3						
Seals edges and removes air pockets	3						
Folds back corner tab	3						
10. Brings final corner up and over top	3						
Seals edges and removes air pockets	3						
Tucks under pocket of previous folds	3						
Leaves small corner exposed for tab	3						

Name _____

12:4A (cont.)

Wrapping Items for Autoclaving	Points Possible	Peer Check		Final Check*		Points Earned**	Comments
		Yes	No	Yes	No		
11. Secures with tape and/or autoclave indicator	3						
12. Labels with date, contents, and size if necessary	3						
13. Wraps with plastic or paper autoclave bag:							
Selects or cuts correct size	2						
Labels wrap or bag correctly	2						
Places clean item inside	2						
Double folds open end(s)	2						
Tapes or seals with heat	2						
14. Checks wrap carefully	3						
15. Replaces all equipment	2						
16. Removes gloves and washes hands	3						
Totals	100						

* Final Check: Instructor or authorized person evaluates.
** Points Earned: Points possible times each "yes" check.

Name _____ Date _____

Evaluated by _____

DIRECTIONS: Practice sterilizing with an autoclave according to the criteria listed. When you are ready for your final check, give this sheet to your instructor.

PROFICIENT

Loading and Operating an Autoclave	Points Possible	Peer Check Yes	No	Final Check* Yes	No	Points Earned**	Comments
1. Assembles equipment and supplies	3						
2. Washes hands and dries thoroughly	3						
3. Checks plug and cord	3						
4. Fills reservoir with distilled water	4						
5. Checks pressure for zero	4						
6. Opens door properly	4						
7. Loads correctly:							
Separates items for same time and temperature	2						
Positions packages on sides	2						
Places basins on sides	2						
Leaves space between items	2						
Checks that no item is in contact with chamber sides, top, or door	2						
8. Fills chamber with correct amount of water	3						
Stops water flow at correct time	3						
9. Checks load	2						
10. Closes and locks door	3						
11. Pulls on door to check	3						
12. Sets control valve to allow temperature and pressure to increase	4						
13. Checks chart to determine time and temperature	4						
14. When temperature and pressure are correct, sets controls to maintain desired temperature	4						
15. Sets timer for correct time—moves past 10 minutes first	4						
16. Checks gauges at intervals	4						
17. Puts on safety glasses	4						

12:4B (cont.)

Loading and Operating an Autoclave	Points Possible	Peer Check		Final Check*		Points Earned**	Comments
		Yes	No	Yes	No		
18. When required time complete, sets controls so autoclave vents the steam from the chamber	4						
19. Allows steam discharge	4						
20. Checks pressure for zero	4						
21. Opens door 1/2 to 1 inch for drying	4						
22. Removes contents when dry and cool	3						
23. Leaves on vent for reuse	3						
24. Turns off if last load	3						
25. Replaces equipment	3						
26. Washes hands	3						
Totals	100						

* Final Check: Instructor or authorized person evaluates.
** Points Earned: Points possible times each "yes" check.

CHAPTER 12:5 USING CHEMICALS FOR DISINFECTION

ASSIGNMENT SHEET

Grade _____   Name _____

INTRODUCTION: You may be required to use chemicals for aseptic control in many health fields. This assignment will help you review the main facts.

INSTRUCTIONS: In the space provided, print the word(s) that best completes the statement or answers the question.

1. Many chemicals do not kill _____ and _____. The appropriate term is
   _____ because _____ does not occur.

2. List three (3) items usually disinfected with chemicals.

3. List two (2) reasons why it is important to thoroughly wash, rinse, and dry all items before placing them in a chemical solution.

4. List five (5) examples of chemical solutions.

5. List two (2) reasons why the manufacturer's directions should be read completely before using any solution.

6. What is the purpose of anti-rust tablets or solutions?

   Can they be added to all chemical solutions? Why or why not?

7. Why should the chemical solution cover the item completely?

8. While the articles are in the solution, a/an _____ should be placed on the container.

9. Where should instruments be stored after being removed from the solution?

10. When should the chemical solutions be changed or discarded?

Name _____ Date _____

Evaluated by _____

DIRECTIONS: Practice using chemicals for disinfection according to the criteria listed. When you are ready for your final check, give this sheet to your instructor.

PROFICIENT

Using Chemicals for Disinfection	Points Possible	Peer Check Yes	No	Final Check* Yes	No	Points Earned**	Comments
1. Assembles equipment and supplies	4						
2. Washes hands and puts on gloves	4						
3. Washes articles thoroughly	4						
Brushes serrated edges	4						
Rinses articles in cool, then hot water	4						
Dries thoroughly	4						
4. Checks container for tight-fitting lid	5						
5. Loads properly:							
Leaves space between items	5						
Leaves hinged instruments open	5						
6. Reads manufacturer's instructions for directions on use of chemical solution	5						
Adds anti-rust substance if needed	3						
7. Pours solution over items to correct depth	5						
Reads label three times: before, during, and after pouring	5						
8. Puts lid on container	5						
9. Removes gloves and washes hands	5						
10. Checks bottle label to determine time required for disinfecting action	5						
11. Leaves instruments in solution for recommended time	5						
12. Washes hands before removing items	5						
13. Uses sterile transfer forceps to place items on sterile towel to dry	5						
14. Stores in dust-free drawer or cabinet	5						
15. Replaces equipment	4						
16. Washes hands	4						
Totals	100						

* Final Check: Instructor or authorized person evaluates.
** Points Earned: Points possible times each "yes" check.

CHAPTER 12:6 CLEANING WITH AN ULTRASONIC UNIT

ASSIGNMENT SHEET

Grade _____   Name _____

INTRODUCTION: Many health facilities use ultrasonic cleaning for instruments and equipment that do not penetrate body tissues. This assignment will help you review the main facts.

INSTRUCTIONS: Read the information on Cleaning with an Ultrasonic Unit. In the space provided, print the word(s) that best completes the statement or answers the question.

1. The ultrasonic unit cleans with _____ waves.

2. Explain *cavitation*.

3. Does ultrasonic cleaning remove all organisms and pathogens? Why or why not?

4. List two (2) reasons why it is important to read the labels carefully before using any cleaning solution.

5. Why should you avoid getting the solutions on the skin?

6. What solution is usually used in the permanent tank?

7. How should the beakers or pans be positioned in the permanent tank?

8. What must be done to all articles before cleaning them in the ultrasonic unit?

9. List two (2) types of jewelry that should not be cleaned in an ultrasonic unit.

10. When a white opaque coating appears on the bottom of the glass beakers, what do you do with the beakers?

11. How is the main tank cleaned?

12. How do you determine the length of time required for cleaning?

Name _____ Date _____

Evaluated by _____

DIRECTIONS: Practice cleaning with an ultrasonic unit according to the criteria listed. When you are ready for your final check, give this sheet to your instructor.

PROFICIENT

Cleaning with an Ultrasonic Unit	Points Possible	Peer Check Yes	No	Final Check* Yes	No	Points Earned**	Comments
1. Assembles equipment and supplies	4						
2. Washes hands and puts on gloves if indicated	4						
3. Cleans articles with brush	4						
4. Rinses articles thoroughly	4						
5. Checks amount of solution in main tank	5						
6. Selects proper solution	5						
7. Places beaker in tank	4						
8. Adjusts beaker band	4						
9. Checks bottom of beaker to be sure it is below level of solution in permanent tank	4						
10. Checks that articles are covered with solution	4						
11. Uses auxiliary pan correctly	5						
12. Checks chart for time	5						
13. Sets timer properly (after turning it past 5)	5						
14. Checks that unit is working by checking for cavitation bubbles	5						
15. When timer signals, removes articles with transfer forceps	4						
16. Places articles on towel	4						
17. Rinses articles thoroughly	4						
18. Checks cleanliness	4						
19. Cleans unit properly:							
Sets container in place	2						
Opens drain valve	2						
Wipes tank with damp cloth or a disinfectant	2						

Cleaning with an Ultrasonic Unit	Points Possible	Peer Check Yes	No	Final Check* Yes	No	Points Earned**	Comments
20. Cleans beakers and pans:							
Empties solution	2						
Washes thoroughly	2						
Rinses completely	2						
Discards etched beakers	2						
21. Replaces equipment	4						
22. Removes gloves if worn and washes hands	4						
Totals	100						

* Final Check: Instructor or authorized person evaluates.
** Points Earned: Points possible times each "yes" check.

CHAPTER 12:7 USING STERILE TECHNIQUES

ASSIGNMENT SHEET

Grade _____   Name _____

INTRODUCTION: Following correct sterile technique is essential in many different procedures. This sheet will help stress the main facts.

INSTRUCTIONS: Read the information on Using Sterile Techniques. In the space provided, print the word(s) that best completes the statement or answers the question.

1. Define *sterile*.

   Define *contaminated*.

2. How can you avoid allowing sterile articles to touch the skin or clothing?

3. What part of a sterile field or tray is considered to be contaminated?

4. List three (3) methods for removing sterile articles from wraps and placing them on a sterile field or tray. Briefly describe each method.

5. Why must a sterile field be kept dry?

6. What should you do if you spill solution on a sterile field?

7. What part of sterile gloves are considered contaminated?

8. Before applying the sterile gloves, you must make sure what has been done in relation to the sterile tray?

9. Once gloves have been applied, where should you hold your hands to avoid contamination?

10. What should you do if you suspect an article is contaminated?

Name _____ Date _____

Evaluated by _____

DIRECTIONS: Practice opening sterile packages according to the criteria listed. When you are ready for your final check, give this sheet to your instructor.

Opening Sterile Packages	Points Possible	Peer Check Yes	No	Final Check* Yes	No	Points Earned**	Comments
1. Assembles equipment and supplies	4						
2. Washes hands	4						
3. Checks date and autoclave indicator on package	6						
4. Keeps work area free of all articles	5						
5. Holds package with point of top flap directed toward body	3						
Loosens fastener	3						
Grasps distal flap	3						
Pulls back and away	3						
Reaches in from side	3						
Allows no contamination	4						
6. Opens first side flap:							
Reaches in from side	3						
Pulls laterally	3						
Allows no contamination	4						
7. Opens second side flap:							
Reaches in from side	3						
Pulls laterally	3						
Allows no contamination	4						
8. Opens proximal edge:							
Pulls toward body	3						
Puts over hand/table	3						
Allows no contamination	4						
9. Transfers item with correct drop technique	8						
10. Transfers item with correct mitten technique	8						
11. Transfers item with correct transfer forcep technique	8						
12. Cleans and replaces all equipment	4						
13. Washes hands	4						
Totals	100						

* Final Check: Instructor or authorized person evaluates.
** Points Earned: Points possible times each "yes" check.

Name _____ Date _____

Evaluated by _____

DIRECTIONS: Practice preparing a sterile dressing tray according to the criteria listed. When you are ready for your final check, give this sheet to your instructor.

PROFICIENT

Preparing a Sterile Dressing Tray	Points Possible	Peer Check Yes	No	Final Check* Yes	No	Points Earned**	Comments
1. Assembles equipment and supplies	3						
2. Washes hands	3						
3. Checks date and autoclave indicator on supplies	4						
4. Opens sterile towel package:							
Unwraps correctly	3						
Picks up by outside	3						
Places on tray correctly	3						
Allows no contamination	4						
Fanfolds back edge	3						
5. Unwraps basin correctly	3						
Places on towel	3						
Allows no contamination	4						
6. Unwraps cotton balls or gauze sponges	3						
Drops into basin	3						
Allows no contamination	4						
7. Unwraps outer dressing	3						
Places on tray correctly	3						
Allows no contamnination	3						
8. Unwraps inner dressing	3						
Places on top of outer dressing correctly	3						
Allows no contamination	3						
9. Adds antiseptic solution:							
Places lid open –side up	3						
Pours off initial flow	3						
Pours into basin without splashing	3						
Allows no contamination	3						
10. Checks tray to make sure all supplies present	3						

12:7B (cont.)

Preparing a Sterile Dressing Tray	Points Possible	Peer Check		Final Check*		Points Earned**	Comments
		Yes	No	Yes	No		
11. Covers with towel:							
Handles outside only	3						
Keeps hands to sides of tray	3						
Unfolds fanfold on towel and covers tray	3						
Allows no contamination	3						
12. Remains with tray at all times	3						
13. Replaces equipment	3						
14. Washes hands	3						
Totals	100						

* Final Check: Instructor or authorized person evaluates.
** Points Earned: Points possible times each "yes" check.

Name _____ Date _____

Evaluated by _____

DIRECTIONS: Practice donning and removing sterile gloves according to the criteria listed. When you are ready for your final check, give this sheet to your instructor.

PROFICIENT

Donning and Removing Sterile Gloves	Points Possible	Peer Check Yes	No	Final Check* Yes	No	Points Earned**	Comments
1. Assembles supplies	4						
2. Checks date and autoclave indicator	4						
3. Washes and dries hands and removes rings	4						
4. Opens outer wrap without contamination	4						
5. Opens inner wrap:							
Handles only outside of wrap	3						
Maintains sterility of wrap and gloves	3						
Positions with cuffs close to body	3						
6. Dons first glove correctly:							
Grasps inside of cuff with thumb and forefinger	3						
Lifts out	3						
Inserts hand	3						
Holds away from body	3						
Avoids counters, and so forth	3						
Maintains sterility of glove	4						
7. Dons second glove correctly:							
Puts gloved hand under cuff	3						
Lifts out	3						
Inserts hand	3						
Maintains sterility of gloves	4						
8. Straightens cuffs:							
Puts gloved hand under cuff, pulls out and up	3						
Maintains sterility of both gloves	4						
9. Interlaces fingers to position gloves without contaminating gloves	4						
10. Handles only sterile items with gloved hands	4						

Donning and Removing Sterile Gloves	Points Possible	Peer Check		Final Check*		Points Earned**	Comments
		Yes	No	Yes	No		
11. Removes gloves correctly:							
Removes first glove by grasping outside with the other gloved hand	4						
Pulls glove down over hand	4						
Removes second glove by placing the ungloved hand inside the cuff	4						
Pulls glove down over hand	4						
Pulls gloves inside out while removing	4						
Puts contaminated gloves in infectious-waste container	4						
12. Washes hands immediately	4						
Totals	100						

* Final Check: Instructor or authorized person evaluates.
** Points Earned: Points possible times each "yes" check.

Name _____ Date _____

Evaluated by _____

DIRECTIONS: Practice changing a sterile dressing according to criteria listed. When you are ready for your final check, give this sheet to your instructor.

PROFICIENT

Changing a Sterile Dressing	Points Possible	Peer Check Yes	No	Final Check* Yes	No	Points Earned**	Comments
1. Checks order or obtains proper authorization	3						
2. Assembles equipment/supplies and checks autoclave indicators and dates	3						
3. Washes hands	3						
4. Prepares sterile tray or obtains commercially prepared kit	3						
5. Introduces self, identifies patient, and explains procedure	3						
6. Provides privacy for patient	3						
7. Prepares tape	3						
8. Positions infectious waste bag correctly	3						
9. Puts on disposable nonsterile gloves	3						
10. Removes dressing:							
Removes tape	3						
Removes dressing carefully	3						
Places tape and dressing in infectious waste bag	3						
11. Checks incision for type, amount, and color of drainage	4						
12. Removes gloves and washes hands	3						
13. Opens sterile tray without contamination	4						
14. Dons sterile gloves correctly	4						
15. Cleanses wound:							
Uses circular motion	3						
Starts at center and moves out	3						
Discards cotton ball or gauze sponge	3						
Does not clean wound without specific order	3						
Goes top to bottom if cleans wound	3						
16. Applies inner dressing	3						

Changing a Sterile Dressing	Points Possible	Peer Check		Final Check*		Points Earned**	Comments
		Yes	No	Yes	No		
17. Applies outer dressing	3						
18. Removes sterile gloves correctly and discards in infectious waste bag	4						
19. Washes hands immediately	3						
20. Applies tape correctly:							
Uses proper length and width	3						
Applies in direction opposite of body movement	3						
21. Checks patient before leaving area	3						
22. Tapes/ties infectious-waste bag securely	3						
23. Replaces equipment	3						
24. Washes hands immediately	3						
25. Records or reports required information	3						
Totals	100						

* Final Check: Instructor or authorized person evaluates.
** Points Earned: Points possible times each "yes" check.

CHAPTER 12:8 MAINTAINING TRANSMISSION-BASED ISOLATION PRECAUTIONS

ASSIGNMENT SHEET

Grade _____ Name _____

INTRODUCTION: Transmission-based isolation techniques will vary from area to area but the same principles are observed in all types. This sheet will help you review these main principles.

INSTRUCTIONS: Read the text information Maintaining Transmission-Based Isolation. In the space provided, print the word(s) that best completes the statement or answers the question.

1. Define *transmission-based isolation*.
   A method or technique of caring for patients who have communicable diseases.

2. What is the difference between standard precautions and transmission-based isolation techniques?
   – Standard precautions: used on all ~~disea~~ patients
   – transmission: used to provide extra protection against specific diseases or pathogens to prevent their spread

3. What is a communicable disease?
   Disease caused by a pathogenic organism that can be easily transmitted to others.

4. List three (3) ways communicable diseases are spread.
   1) Direct contact w/ the patient
   2) Contact w/ dirty linen, equipment, and/or supplies
   3) Contact w/ blood, body fluids, secretions, and excretions

5. Identify three (3) factors that help determine what type of isolation is used.
   1) The causitive organism of the disease
   2) the way the organism is transmitted
   3) weather or not the pathogen is antibiotic resistant

6. Define *contaminated*.
   Objects contain disease producing organisms

   Define *clean*.
   Objects don't contain disease producing organisms.

7. Using the guidelines established by the Centers for Disease Control and Prevention (CDC), place the letter or letters for the type of isolation used in Column B by any statement in Column A that pertains to this type of isolation.

	Column A		Column B
A	1. Used for measles and tuberculosis	A.	Airborne
C	2. Used for pneumonia, pertussis, and severe viral infections	B.	Contact
D	3. Used for all patients	C.	Droplet
B	4. Gloves must be worn when entering room	D.	Standard
ABCD	5. Uses standard precautions		
B	6. Used for wound infections caused by multidrug-resistant organisms		
A	7. Anyone entering room must wear high-efficiency particulate air (HEPA) mask		
C	8. Masks must be worn when working within three feet of patient		
A	9. Used for pathogens transmitted by airborne droplet nuclei		
B	10. Room and items in it should receive daily cleaning and disinfection		
B C A	11. Patient should be placed in a private room		
C A	12. Used for pathogens transmitted by large particle droplets		
A	13. Room air should be discharged to outdoor air or filtered		
B A C	14. Patient must wear a mask appropriate for the disease if transport from room is necessary		

8. What is protective or reverse isolation?

Method used to protect patients from organisms present in the environment.

9. List two (2) types of patients who may require protective or reverse isolation.

1) Severely burned patients
2) patients recieving chemotherapy or radiation

10. List four (4) precautions that may be required for protective or reverse isolation.

1) clean, disinf. room
2) filters
3) sterile

Name _____ Date _____

Evaluated by _____

DIRECTIONS: Practice donning and removing transmission-based isolation garments according to the criteria listed. When you are ready for your final check, give this sheet to your instructor.

PROFICIENT

Donning and Removing Transmission-Based Isolation Garments	Points Possible	Peer Check Yes	No	Final Check* Yes	No	Points Earned**	Comments
1. Assembles equipment and supplies	4						
2. Washes hands	4						
3. Removes rings	4						
4. Places watch in plastic bag or on paper towel	4						
5. Applies mask correctly:							
Handles very little	2						
Covers mouth and nose	2						
Ties in back securely	2						
Changes mask every 30 minutes or anytime it gets wet	2						
6. Rolls up uniform sleeves	3						
7. Puts on gown correctly:							
Keeps hands inside shoulders	2						
Works arms in gently	2						
Adjusts neck with hands inside neck band	2						
Ties at neck first	2						
Ties at waist	2						
Handles only inside of gown	3						
8. Applies gloves correctly	3						
Covers cuffs of gown with gloves	3						
Removal of Garments:							
9. Unties waist ties of gown first	3						
10. Removes gloves:							
Uses gloved hand to grasp outside of opposite glove	2						
Pulls glove off inside out	2						
Places ungloved hand under cuff to remove second glove	2						

Donning and Removing Transmission-Based Isolation Garments	Points Possible	Peer Check Yes	No	Final Check* Yes	No	Points Earned**	Comments
Pulls glove off inside out	2						
Places gloves in infectious waste container	2						
11. Washes hands thoroughly	3						
Operates faucet with towel	3						
12. Removes mask after gloves	2						
Handles ties only	2						
Places in infectious waste container	2						
13. Removes gown last	2						
Unties neck ties	2						
Places one hand inside cuff and pulls sleeve over hand	2						
Places covered hand on outside of gown to pull gown sleeve over second hand	2						
Eases out of gown gently	2						
Folds gown so inside of gown is on outside	2						
Rolls gown	2						
Places gown in linen hamper (or infectious-waste can if gown disposable)	2						
Touches only inside of gown	3						
14. Washes hands thoroughly	3						
15. Removes watch by touching only inside of plastic bag or top part of towel	2						
16. Opens door with towel, discards towel in waste can	2						
17. Washes hands immediately	3						
Totals	100						

* Final Check: Instructor or authorized person evaluates.
** Points Earned: Points possible times each "yes" check.

Name _____ Date _____

Evaluated by _____

DIRECTIONS: Practice working in a transmission-based isolation unit according to the criteria listed.for your final check give this sheet to your instructor. When you are ready for your final check give this sheet to your instructor.

PROFICIENT

Working in a Hospital Transmission-Based Isolation Unit	Points Possible	Peer Check Yes	No	Final Check* Yes	No	Points Earned**	Comments
1. Assembles equipment and supplies	2						
2. Washes hands	2						
3. Dons isolation garments	2						
4. Records vital signs:							
Tapes paper to door	3						
Keeps watch in plastic bag/paper towel	3						
Writes information on paper without touching paper on door	3						
5. Transfers food correctly:							
Obtains tray inside unit	3						
Receives glasses by bottom	3						
Receives plates from opposite side	3						
Allows no contamination	3						
6. Disposes of food:							
Pours liquids into sink	3						
Flushes soft liquids in toilet	3						
Places hard solids in waste container	3						
Places disposable utensils/dishes in trash	3						
Cleans metal utensils	3						
7. Handles linens:							
Folds and rolls	3						
Places in linen bag	3						
Folds down top edge	3						
Tells clean person to cuff outside of infectious-waste laundry bag	3						
Places linens in outside bag	3						
Allows no contamination	3						
Tells clean person how to label and tie final bag	3						
8. Disposes of trash:							
Ties plastic bag shut	3						
Places in cuffed outer biohazardous-waste bag	3						
Allows no contamination during transfer	3						
Tells clean person how to tape or tie and label outer bag	3						

Working in a Hospital Transmission-Based Isolation Unit	Points Possible	Peer Check Yes	No	Final Check* Yes	No	Points Earned**	Comments
9. Transfers equipment:							
Cleans and disinfects thoroughly inside unit	3						
Places in bag	3						
Seals top of bag	3						
Places in cuffed outer infectious-waste bag without contamination	3						
Tells clean person how to seal, tape, and label outer bag	3						
10. Checks patient before leaving unit	3						
Offers bedpan/urinal	3						
11. Removes isolation garments correctly	2						
12. Washes hands	2						
Totals	100						

* Final Check: Instructor or authorized person evaluates.
** Points Earned: Points possible times each "yes" check.

CHAPTER 13:1 MEASURING AND RECORDING VITAL SIGNS

ASSIGNMENT SHEET

Grade _____   Name _____

INTRODUCTION: Vital signs are important indicators of health states of the body. This assignment will help you review the main facts about vital signs.

INSTRUCTIONS: Read the information on Measuring and Recording Vital Signs. In the space provided, print the word(s) that best completes the statements or answers the questions.

1. Use the Key Terms to complete the crossword puzzle.

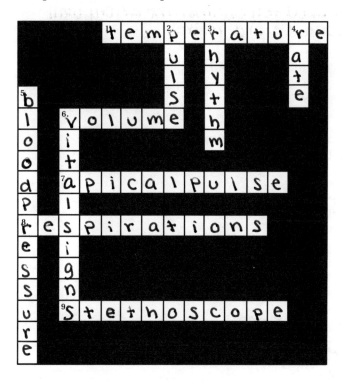

ACROSS

✗ Measurement of the balance between heat lost and heat produced

✗ Strength of the pulse

✗ Pulse taken at the apex of the heart with a stethoscope

✗ Measurement of breaths taken by a patient

✗ Instrument used to take apical pulse

DOWN

✗ Pressure of the blood felt against the wall of an artery

✗ Regularity of the pulse or respirations

✗ Number of beats per minute

✗ Measurement of the force exerted by the heart against arterial walls

✗ Various determinations that provide information about body conditions

---

2. List the four (4) main vital signs.
   1) Temperature   3) Respirations
   2) Pulse   4) Blood Pressure

3. Why is it essential that vital signs are measured accurately?
   Many times they are the first indication of a disease or abnormalty in a patient.

4. Identify four (4) common sites in the body where temperature can be measured.
   1) Oral (mouth)   3) axillary (armpit)
   2) Rectal (rectum) 4) aural (ear)

5. Define *pulse*.
   The pressure of blood felt against the artery wall as the heart contracts and relaxes.

   List three (3) factors recorded about a pulse.
   1) Rate
   2) Rhythm
   3) volume

6. What three (3) factors are noted about respirations?
   1) Respiration count
   2) Rhythm
   3) Character (type)

7. Identify the two (2) readings noted on a blood pressure.
   1) Systolic
   2) Diastolic

8. List three (3) times you may have to take an apical pulse.
   1) illness
   2) hardening of the arteries
   3) weak/rapid pulse
   4) doctors orders

9. What should you do if you note any abnormality or change in any vital sign?
   You must immediately report it to your supervisor.

10. What should you do if you are not able to obtain a correct reading for a vital sign?
    Ask another individual to Check.

11. Convert the following Fahrenheit (F) temperatures to Celsius (C) temperatures. Use the formula: $C = (F - 32) \times 5/9$ or 0.5556.

For example: F is equal to $120°$. What is Celsius?

Subtract 32 from F: $120 - 32 = 88$

Multiply answer by 5/9 or 0.5556: $88 \times 0.5556 = 48.8928$ or 48.9

Celsius temperature is $48.9°$.

Note: Round off answers to nearest tenth or one decimal point.

a. 140° F **60°C**

b. 70° F **21.11°C**

c. 50° F **10°C**

d. 38° F **3.33°C**

e. 86° F **30°C**

f. 105° F **40.55°C**

g. 138° F **58.88°C**

h. 204° F **95.55°C**

i. 99.6° F **37.55°C**

j. 25° F **-3.88°C**

12. Convert the following Celsius (C) temperatures to Fahrenheit (F) temperatures. Use the formula: $F = (C \times 9/5$ or $1.8) + 32$

For example: C is equal to $22°$. What is Fahrenheit (F)?

Multiply C by 9/5 or 1.8: $22 \times 1.8 = 39.6$

Add 32 to the answer: $39.6 + 32 = 71.6$

Fahrenheit temperature is $71.6°$.

Note: Round off answers to nearest tenth or one decimal point.

a. 32° C **89.6°F**

b. 54° C **129.2°F**

c. 8° C **46.4°F**

d. 91° C **195.8°F**

e. 0° C **32°F**

f. 72° C **161.6°F**

g. 26° C **78.8°F**

h. 81° C **177.8°F**

i. 99.8° C **211.64°F**

j. 46.1° C **114.98°F**

CHAPTER 13:2 MEASURING AND RECORDING TEMPERATURE

ASSIGNMENT SHEET

Grade _____ Name _____

INTRODUCTION: In addition to being able to take temperatures, it will be important for you to know the main facts about body temperature. This assignment will help you review these facts.

INSTRUCTIONS: Read the information on Measuring and Recording Temperature. In the space provided, print the word(s) that best completes the statements or answers the questions.

1. Define *temperature*.
   The balance between heat loss and the heat produced by the body.

2. List three main reasons why temperature may vary.
   1) Individuals have different body temperatures
   2) Time of day
   3) Location of where the temperature is taken

3. The normal range for body temperature is ___*97*___ to ___*100*___ degrees.

4. A normal oral temperature is ___*98.6*___ degrees. The clinical thermometer is left in place for ___*3-5*___ minutes.

5. A normal rectal temperature is ___*99.6*___ degrees. The clinical thermometer is left in place for ___*3-5*___ minutes.

6. A normal axillary temperature is ___*97.6*___ degrees. The clinical thermometer is left in place for ___*10*___ minutes.

7. What is the most accurate method for taking a temperature? Why?
   The rectal measurement is most accurate because it is an internal measurement.

8. What is the least accurate method for taking a temperature? Why?
   The axillary and groin measurements because they are external measurements.

9. What is an aural temperature?
   It is a measurement taken with a special thermometer in the ear or auditory canal.

   How does an aural thermometer measure temperature?
   It detects and measures the thermal infared energy radiating from blood vessels in the tympanic membrane.

10. What is the difference between hyperthermia and hypothermia?
   - <u>Hyperthermia</u>: when the body temperature exceeds 104°F measured rectally
   - <u>Hypothermia</u>: when the body temperature is below 96°F measured rectally

11. List two (2) ways you can tell a rectal clinical thermometer from an oral clinical thermometer.
   - <u>oral</u>- shorter, rounder bulb w/ blue tip
   - <u>rectal</u>- short, stubby, rounded bulb w/ red tip
   - *sometimes oral or rectal is written on the tip*

12. Briefly describe the proper procedure for cleanup and disposal of a broken clinical thermometer.
   - never use a vacuum cleaner
   - never pour mercury down a drain or down the toilet
   - close doors + other indoor areas
   - open the windows in the room with the spill
   - put on gloves
   - use two cards or stiff paper to push the droplets of mercury and broken glass into a container w/ a tight fitting lid
   - use an eyedropper to pick up the balls necessary
   - use a flashlight to find the beads
   - wipe the entire area with a damp sponge
   - place all cleanup material in a plastic container labeled Mercury for recycling

13. How can you prevent cross-contamination while using the probe of an electronic thermometer?
   use a disposable cover before the temperature is taken

14. How do plastic or paper thermometers register body temperature?
   Chemical dots/strips change color when exposed to certain temperatures.

15. Why is it important to ask patients if they have had anything to eat or drink or if they have smoked before taking an oral temperature?
   It could alter the temperature reading

16. How long should a thermometer soak in a disinfectant (after cleaning) before it is safe to rinse in cold water and use on a patient?
   30 minutes

READING A THERMOMETER

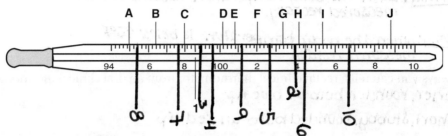

17. After the following steps is a list of temperatures that are to be recorded along the bottom of the illustrated thermometer:

    * Each temperature reading is preceded by a listed number (1, 2, 3, etc.).

    * Locate the line on the sketch that reflects the temperature reading.

    * Draw an arrow to the correct line on the thermometer.

    * Place the listed number below the arrow (1, 2, 3, etc.).

    * See Example 1.

    1. 98^6 (Example)

    2. 100^4

    3. 99

    4. 99^8

    5. 102^6

    6. 104^4

    7. 97^6

    8. 95^4

    9. 101^2

    10. 106^8

18. Note that in the previous sketch, letters appear along the top of the thermometer. Each letter has an arrow pointing to a line on the thermometer. This is the temperature reading. Record each reading beside the corresponding letter that follows. (Note Example A.)

    A. 95 (Example)

    B. 96.2

    C. 98

    D. 100.1

    E. 100.4

    F. 102

    G. 103.2

    H. 104.1

    I. 105.2

    J. 108.4

Name _____ Date _____

Evaluated by _____

DIRECTIONS: Practice cleaning a clinical thermometer according to the criteria listed. When you are ready f
your final check, give this sheet to your instructor.

PROFICIENT

Cleaning a Clinical Thermometer	Points Possible	Peer Check Yes	No	Final Check* Yes	No	Points Earned**	Comments
1. Assembles equipment and supplies	5						
2. Washes hands and puts on gloves if indicated	5						
3. Wipes thermometer from top to bulb with soapy cotton ball	7						
4. Rinses in cool water	7						
5. Shakes down correctly:							
Holds securely	5						
Uses snapping motion of wrist	5						
Shakes down to 96° F (35.6° C)	5						
6. Places in container of disinfectant	7						
7. Removes gloves and washes hands	6						
8. Soaks thermometer at least 30 minutes	7						
9. Wipes with alcohol cotton ball after soaking	6						
10. Rinses in cool water	6						
11. Checks for signs of breakage	7						
12. Reads to be sure it is 96° F (35.6°C) or less	7						
13. Places clean thermometer in clean gauze-lined container	5						
14. Replaces all equipment used	5						
15. Washes hands	5						
Totals	100						

* Final Check: Instructor or authorized person evaluates.
** Points Earned: Points possible times each "yes" check.

Name _____ Date _____

Evaluated by _____

DIRECTIONS: Practice measuring and recording an oral temperature according to the criteria listed. When you are ready for your final check, give this sheet to your instructor.

		Peer Check		Final Check*			
Measuring and Recording Oral Temperature	**Points Possible**	**PROFICIENT** **Yes**	**No**	**Yes**	**No**	**Points Earned***	**Comments**
1. Assembles equipment and supplies	4						
2. Washes hands and puts on gloves	5						
3. Introduces self and identifies patient	4						
4. Explains procedure	4						
5. Questions patient on eating, drinking, or smoking	6						
6. Wipes thermometer	4						
7. Checks and reads thermometer and applies sheath if used	6						
8. Instructs patient on holding it in mouth	6						
9. Cautions against biting thermometer	6						
10. Leaves in place 3 to 5 minutes	6						
11. Removes and wipes or removes sheath, and holds at stem end for reading	6						
12. Reads to nearest two-tenths of a degree	8						
13. Records correctly	8						
14. Cleans correctly:							
Wipes with soapy cotton ball	3						
Rinses in cool water	3						
Shakes down correctly	3						
Soaks proper time	3						
15. Replaces all equipment	4						
16. Removes gloves and washes hands	5						
17. Recognizes an abnormal reading and reports it immediately	6						
Totals	100						

* Final Check: Instructor or authorized person evaluates.
** Points Earned: Points possible times each "yes" check.

Name _____ Date _____

Evaluated by _____

DIRECTIONS: Practice measuring and recording a rectal temperature according to the criteria listed. When you are ready for your final check, give this sheet to your instructor.

PROFICIENT

Measuring and Recording Rectal Temperature	Points Possible	Peer Check Yes	No	Final Check* Yes	No	Points Earned**	Comments
1. Assembles equipment and supplies	4						
2. Washes hands and puts on gloves	4						
3. Introduces self, identifies patient, and explains procedure	4						
4. Provides privacy for the patient	4						
5. Checks and reads thermometer and applies sheath if used	5						
6. Places lubricant on tissue and rolls bulb end of thermometer in lubricant	5						
7. Positions patient on side	4						
8. Folds back covers to expose anal area	5						
9. Explains procedure to patient while inserting thermometer	4						
10. Inserts thermometer 1 to 1½ inches in rectum (½ to 1 inch for infant)	5						
11. Replaces bed covers while holding thermometer in place	4						
12. Holds in place 3 to 5 minutes	5						
13. Removes thermometer and explains action to patient	4						
14. Wipes off excess lubricant with tissue, or removes sheath if used, and holds at stem end for reading	5						
15. Reads to nearest two-tenths of a degree	8						
16. Records correctly and places (R) by reading	8						
17. Repositions patient	4						
18. Cleans thermometer correctly	4						
19. Replaces equipment	4						
20. Removes gloves and washes hands	4						
21. Recognizes an abnormal reading and reports it immediately	6						
Totals	100						

* Final Check: Instructor or authorized person evaluates.
** Points Earned: Points possible times each "yes" check.

Name _____ Date _____

Evaluated by _____

DIRECTIONS: Practice measuring and recording an axillary temperature according to the criteria listed. When you are ready for your final check, give this sheet to your instructor.

PROFICIENT

Measuring and Recording Axillary Temperature	Points Possible	Peer Check		Final Check*		Points Earned**	Comments
		Yes	No	Yes	No		
1. Assembles equipment and supplies	5						
2. Washes hands and puts on gloves if needed	5						
3. Introduces self and identifies patient	5						
4. Explains procedure	5						
5. Wipes thermometer	5						
6. Checks and reads thermometer and applies sheath if used	6						
7. Dries axillary area	6						
8. Positions thermometer correctly with arm over chest	6						
9. Leaves in place 10 minutes	7						
10. Removes and wipes, or removes sheath, and holds at stem end for reading	6						
11. Reads to nearest two-tenths of a degree	8						
12. Records correctly and places (Ax) by reading	8						
13. Repositions patient for comfort and safety	6						
14. Cleans thermometer correctly	6						
15. Replaces equipment	5						
16. Removes gloves if worn and washes hands	5						
17. Recognizes an abnormal reading and reports it immediately	6						
Totals	100						

* Final Check: Instructor or authorized person evaluates.
** Points Earned: Points possible times each "yes" check.

Name _____ Date _____

Evaluated by _____

DIRECTIONS: Practice measuring and recording a tympanic (aural) temperature according to the criteria listed. When you are ready for your final check, give this sheet to your instructor.

PROFICIENT

Measuring and Recording a Tympanic (Aural) Temperature	Points Possible	Peer Check Yes	No	Final Check* Yes	No	Points Earned**	Comments
1. Assembles equipment and supplies	3						
2. Washes hands and puts on gloves if needed	4						
3. Introduces self and identifies patient	4						
4. Explains procedure	4						
5. Removes thermometer from base and selects proper mode	5						
6. Installs probe cover correctly	5						
7. Checks that thermometer indicates "ready" with correct mode	5						
8. Positions patient correctly with easy access to ear	4						
9. Pulls ear pinna back:							
Pulls straight back for infant under 1 year	4						
Pulls up and back for children and adults	4						
10. Inserts probe into ear canal and seals canal	5						
11. Presses scan or activator button	5						
12. Holds thermometer steady for 1 or 2 seconds or time required	5						
13. Removes probe from ear	5						
14. Reads temperature correctly	7						
15. Records correctly and places (T) by reading	7						
16. Removes and discards probe cover correctly	4						
17. Returns thermometer to base unit	4						
18. Repositions patient for comfort and safety	4						
19. Replaces all equipment	3						
20. Removes gloves if worn and washes hands	4						
21. Recognizes an abnormal reading and reports it immediately	5						
Totals	100						

* Final Check: Instructor or authorized person evaluates.
** Points Earned: Points possible times each "yes" check.

Name _____ Date _____

Evaluated by _____

DIRECTIONS: Practice measuring and recording temperature with an electronic thermometer according to the criteria listed. When you are ready for your final check, give this sheet to your instructor.

PROFICIENT

Measuring Temperature with an Electronic Thermometer	Points Possible	Peer Check		Final Check*		Points Earned**	Comments
		Yes	No	Yes	No		
1. Assembles equipment and supplies	4						
2. Washes hands and puts on gloves if indicated	5						
3. Introduces self and identifies patient	4						
4. Explains procedure	4						
5. Positions patient correctly and questions patient on eating, drinking, or smoking for oral temperature	7						
6. If necessary, inserts probe into thermometer unit and turns unit on	6						
7. Covers probe with sheath or probe cover	6						
8. Inserts probe into desired location and holds probe in position	7						
9. Removes probe when thermometer signals that temperature has been recorded	7						
10. Reads thermometer correctly	8						
11. Records correctly	8						
12. Removes and discards sheath or probe cover correctly	6						
13. Repositions patient for comfort and safety	6						
14. If necessary, positions probe in correct storage position in thermometer unit and turns unit off	6						
15. Replaces all equipment	4						
16. Removes gloves if worn and washes hands	5						
17. Recognizes an abnormal reading and reports it immediately	7						
Totals	100						

* Final Check: Instructor or authorized person evaluates.
** Points Earned: Points possible times each "yes" check.

ASSIGNMENT SHEET

Grade _____   Name _____

INTRODUCTION: One of the vital signs you will be required to record is pulse. This assignment sheet will assist you in learning the sites for taking pulse and the important aspects about pulse.

INSTRUCTIONS: Read the information about Measuring and Recording Pulse. In the space provided, print the word(s) that best completes the statement or answers the question.

1. Define *pulse*. The pressure of ~~an artery~~ the blood pushing against the wall of an artery as the heart beats + rests.

2. (a) Study the outlined figure. As you identify each pulse site, enter the name beside the corresponding letter on the following list.

   A. Temporal Artery

   B. Carotid Artery

   C. Brachial Artery

   D. Radial Artery

   E. Femoral Artery

   F. Popliteal Artery

   G. Dorsalis Pedis Artery (Pedal Pulse)

   (b) Circle the site (on the sketch) that is used most frequently for taking pulse.

3. The three (3) factors that must be noted about each and every pulse are:
   –age –sex –body size

4. What is the normal pulse range for each of the following?

   a. Adults: 60 – 90 bpm

   b. Children over 7 years old: 70 –90 bpm

   c. Children from 1 to 7 years old: 80 - 110 bpm

   d. Infants: 100 - 160 bpm

5. List three (3) factors that could cause an increase in a pulse rate.
   –exercise –stimulant drugs –fever

6. List three (3) factors that could cause a decrease in a pulse rate.
   –sleep –depressant drugs – coma

7. In an adult, a pulse rate under 60 beats per minute is called Bradycardia. A pulse rate above 100 beats per minute is called Tachycardia. An irregular or abnormal rhythm is a/an arrhythmia.

Name _____ Date _____

Evaluated by _____

DIRECTIONS: Practice measuring and recording pulse according to the criteria listed. When you are ready for your final check, give this sheet to your instructor.

Measuring and Recording Pulse	Points Possible	Peer Check Yes	Peer Check No	Final Check* Yes	Final Check* No	Points Earned**	Comments
PROFICIENT							
1. Assembles supplies	5						
2. Washes hands	5						
3. Introduces self, identifies patient, and explains procedure	6						
4. Positions patient with arm supported and palm down	8						
5. Places fingers correctly over selected pulse site	8						
6. Counts one minute	8						
7. Obtains correct count to ± 2 beats per minute	15						
8. Records accurately	10						
9. Notes rhythm and volume	10						
10. Checks patient before leaving	6						
11. Replaces equipment	5						
12. Washes hands	5						
13. Recognizes an abnormal measurement and reports it immediately	9						
Totals	100						

* Final Check: Instructor or authorized person evaluates.
** Points Earned: Points possible times each "yes" check.

CHAPTER 13:4 MEASURING AND RECORDING RESPIRATIONS

ASSIGNMENT SHEET

Grade _____   Name _____

INTRODUCTION: This assignment will help you review the main facts regarding respirations.

INSTRUCTIONS: Read the information about Measuring and Recording Respirations. In the space provided, print the word(s) that best completes the statement or answers the question.

1. Define *respiration.* The process of taking in oxygen + expelling carbon dioxide.

2. One respiration consists of one _inspiration_ and one _expiration_.

3. What is the normal rate for respirations in adults? 14-18 breaths per minute 12-20

   What is the normal rate for children? 16-25

   What is the normal rate for infants? 30-50

4. List four (4) words to describe the character or volume of respirations.

   1) deep   3) labored

   2) shallow 4) difficult

5. List two (2) words to describe the rhythm of respirations.

   1) regular

   2) irregular

6. Briefly define the following words.

   dyspnea: difficult/labored breathing

   apnea: abscence of respirations (usually temporary)

   Cheyne–Stokes: periods of dyspnea followed by periods of apnea

   rales: bubbling or noisy sounds

   tachypnea: respiratory rate above 25

   bradypnea: slow respiratory rate below 10

   wheezing: difficult breathing ō high pitched whistling sound

7. Why is it important that the patient is not aware that you are counting respirations?
   The patient may breathe slower/faster if they're aware that you're counting respirations.

8. If you are taking a TPR, how can you count respirations without letting the patient know that you are doing it?
   Pretend to be counting pulse.

Name _____ Date _____

Evaluated by _____

DIRECTIONS: Practice measuring and recording respirations according to the criteria listed. When you are ready for your final check, give this sheet to your instructor.

PROFICIENT

Measuring and Recording Respirations	Points Possible	Peer Check Yes	No	Final Check* Yes	No	Points Earned**	Comments
1. Assembles supplies	5						
2. Washes hands	5						
3. Introduces self and identifies patient	5						
4. Positions patient correctly	5						
5. Leaves hand on pulse site	7						
6. Counts 1 minute	7						
7. Keeps patient unaware of counting activity	8						
8. Obtains correct count to ± 1 breath per minute	15						
9. Records correctly	10						
10. Notes rhythm and character	10						
11. Checks patient before leaving	5						
12. Replaces equipment	5						
13. Washes hands	5						
14. Recognizes an abnormal measurement and reports it immediately	8						
Totals	100						

* Final Check: Instructor or authorized person evaluates.
** Points Earned: Points possible times each "yes" check.

CHAPTER 13:5 GRAPHING TPR

ASSIGNMENT SHEET #1

Grade _____ Name _____

INTRODUCTION: This assignment will provide you with practice in graphing TPRs.

INSTRUCTIONS: Use the blank graphic chart to record the following information. Be sure to include the entries that are shown under Notes in this sample case history.

Patient: Louise Simmers   Physician: Dr. James Webber

Room 238   Hospital No.:   534–23

Admitted: 11/1/ ——

Date	Time	T	P	R	Notes
11/1/	12 NOON	98^6	88	20	BP 120/80
	4 PM	98^8	80	22	
11/2/	8 AM	97^4	68	16	BP 124/78
	12 NOON	98^2	74	18	
	4 PM	98^8	86	22	
	8 PM	99	110	28	
11/3/—	8 AM	97^2	64	14	BP 116/78
	12 NOON	Sleeping—not disturbed			
	4 PM	96^8	88	22	
	8 PM	97^4	80	20	
	12 MN	98^2	84	18	
11/4/—	4 AM	98^8	90	22	BP 110/74
	8 AM	99^2	94	24	
	12 NOON	100^4	96	24	
	4 PM	102^6 R	92	24	
	8 PM	102^4 R	90	20	
	12 MN	103^8 R	98	22	
11/5/—	4 AM	104^6 R	110	26	Antibiotics
	8 AM	103^6 R	120	28	BP 124/86
	12 NOON	99^8 R	90	20	
	4 PM	99^6 R	82	18	
	8 PM	99	86	20	
	12 MN	98	84	18	
11/6/—	8 AM	97^6	68	14	BP 108/68
	12 NOON	98^2	72	16	
	4 PM	98^6	76	16	
	8 PM	98^6	110	24	
	12 MN	In OR—Emergency surgery			
11/7/—	8 AM	98	68	20	
	4 PM	98^6	76	18	Discharged to another hospital

GRAPHIC CHART

Family Name		First Name		Attending Physician			Room No.		Hosp. No.	

Date								
Day in Hospital								
Day P O or P P								

	Hour	A M	P M	A M	P M	A M	P M	A M	P M	A M	P M	A M	P M	A M	P M	A M	P M
		4 8 12	4 8 12	4 8 12	4 8 12	4 8 12	4 8 12	4 8 12	4 8 12	4 8 12	4 8 12	4 8 12	4 8 12	4 8 12	4 8 12	4 8 12	4 8 12

TEMPERATURE

106
105
104
103
102
101
100
99 Normal
98
97
96

PULSE

150
140
130
120
110
100
90
80
70
60

RESPIRATION

50
40
30
20
10

Blood Pressure								
Fluid Intake								
Urine								
Defecation								
Weight								

ASSIGNMENT SHEET #2

Grade _____ Name _____

INTRODUCTION: Tamika Petro was admitted to Ram Hospital with an elevated temperature and abdominal pain. This assignment will provide practice in graphing her TPRs.

INSTRUCTIONS: Chart the following information on a TPR graphic chart.

Patient: Tamika Petro   Room: 238

Physician: Dr. John Vaughn   Hospital No.: 36-26-38

Date	Time	T	P	R	Notes
11/8/—	4 PM	104^6 R	128	36	Admission
	8 PM	104^4 R	126	34	BP 134/86
	12 MN	103 R	116	30	
11/9/—	4 AM	99^8 R	86	26	
	8 AM	99 R	88	20	BP 124/76
	12 NOON	103^4 R	108	28	
	4 PM	102^4 R	100	22	
	8 PM	In OR—Appendectomy by Dr. Vaughn			
	12 MN	100^6 Ax	124	28	
11/10/—	4 AM	100^4 Ax	132	24	
	8 AM	97^8 Ax	82	18	BP 110/68
	12 NOON	98	90	16	
	4 PM	99	86	18	
	8 PM	99^6	94	18	
	12 MN	98^8	80	14	
11/11/—	8 AM	98	82	12	BP 106/68
	12 NOON	98^6	90	18	
	4 PM	101^6	106	24	
	8 PM	102^8 R	110	28	
	12 MN	103^3 R	120	34	Antibiotics
11/12/—	4 AM	101^2 R	118	26	
	8 AM	99^6 R	98	18	BP 108/78
	12 NOON	98	86	12	
	4 PM	98^6	80	16	
	8 PM	98	82	20	
11/13/—	8 AM	97	64	12	BP 122/82
	4 PM	96^8	68	16	
11/14/—	8 AM	97^6	60	12	BP 120/78
	4 PM	98^6	86	18	Discharged

GRAPHIC CHART

Family Name		First Name	Attending Physician			Room No.	Hosp. No.

Date								
Day in Hospital								
Day P O or P P								

	Hour	AM / PM	AM / PM	AM / PM	AM / PM	AM / PM	AM / PM	AM / PM	AM / PM
		4 8 12 4 8 12	4 8 12 4 8 12	4 8 12 4 8 12	4 8 12 4 8 12	4 8 12 4 8 12	4 8 12 4 8 12	4 8 12 4 8 12	4 8 12 4 8 12

TEMPERATURE

106
105
104
103
102
101
100
99 Normal
98
97
96

PULSE

150
140
130
120
110
100
90
80
70
60

RESPIRATION

50
40
30
20
10

Blood Pressure								
Fluid Intake								
Urine								
Defecation								
Weight								

CHAPTER 13:5 GRAPHING TPR

ASSIGNMENT SHEET #3

Grade _____   Name _____

INTRODUCTION: This assignment will allow you to improve your skills on graphing TPRs.

INSTRUCTIONS: Chart the following information on a blank graphic chart.

Patient: Ralph Brown   Room: 238

Physician: Dr. Jacoby   Hospital No.:   589-2112

Date	Time	T	P	R	Notes
11/14/—	8 PM	103^4 R	136	38	BP 180/90
	12 MN	103^6 R	130	36	
11/15/—	4 AM	102^4 R	118	28	
	8 AM	104^8 R	120	18	BP 178/88
	12 NOON	106 R	138	28	Antibiotics
	4 PM	105^6 R	140	36	
	8 PM	99^8 R	138	20	
	12 MN	101	110	24	
11/16/—	4 AM	101^8	102	20	
	8 AM	102^6	108	24	BP 172/86
	12 NOON	101^4	102	26	
	4 PM	103 R	120	34	
	8 PM	98^6 R	102	24	
	12 MN	98^8	80	20	
11/17/—	4 AM	97^8	86	18	
	8 AM	98^2	64	12	BP 134/72
	12 NOON	99	74	18	
	4 PM	98^6	110	26	
	8 PM	99^2	86	16	
11/18/—	8 AM	97^2	66	12	
	12 NOON	98^2	78	18	
	4 PM	98^6	86	20	BP 126/88
	8 PM	99^4	82	16	
11/19/—	8 AM	97^2	68	14	BP 124/82
	12 NOON	98^4	86	20	
	4 PM	98^8	80	18	
11/20/—	8 AM	97^8	64	12	BP 120/84
	4 PM	98^4	82	18	
11/21/—	8 AM	98	72	14	Discharged

GRAPHIC CHART

Family Name		First Name		Attending Physician				Room No.		Hosp. No.	

Date							
Day in Hospital							
Day P O or P P							

	Hour	AM / PM 4 8 12 4 8 12	AM / PM 4 8 12 4 8 12	AM / PM 4 8 12 4 8 12	AM / PM 4 8 12 4 8 12	AM / PM 4 8 12 4 8 12	AM / PM 4 8 12 4 8 12	AM / PM 4 8 12 4 8 12	AM / PM 4 8 12 4 8 12
TEMPERATURE	106								
	105								
	104								
	103								
	102								
	101								
	100								
	99 Normal								
	98								
	97								
	96								
PULSE	150								
	140								
	130								
	120								
	110								
	100								
	90								
	80								
	70								
	60								
RESPIRATION	50								
	40								
	30								
	20								
	10								

Blood Pressure								
Fluid Intake								
Urine								
Defecation								
Weight								

ASSIGNMENT SHEET #4

Grade _____   Name _____

INTRODUCTION: The following patient was admitted to Ram Hospital on 11/28/—. Admitted by Dr. Yoder, the diagnosis was mononucleosis. This assignment will give you practice in graphing TPRs.

INSTRUCTIONS: Chart the following information on a blank graphic chart. If you get this graphic 100% correct, you will not have to do graphic #5.

Patient: Roger Daugherty   Room: 238
Weight : 200 lbs   Hospital No.: 555-44

Date	Time	T	P	R	Notes
11/28/—	4 PM	103^6 R	108	30	BP 128/80
	8 PM	104^2 R	100	26	
	12 MN	103^2 R	118	28	Aspirin Gr X
11/29/—	4 AM	101^6 R	100	24	
	8 AM	100^4 R	86	20	BP 124/84
	12 NOON	103^6 R	122	28	Aspirin Gr X
	4 PM	100^2 R	106	22	
	8 PM	104^8 R	110	32	
	12 MN	105^8 R	148	38	
11/30/—	4 AM	99^4 R	88	20	
	8 AM	98^6 R	86	18	BP 118/76
	12 NOON	98^8	80	20	
	4 PM	99^8	94	18	
	8 PM	98^2	84	16	
12/1/—	8 AM	97^6	60	12	BP 130/78
	12 NOON	98^2	66	14	
	4 PM	99^2	82	20	
	8 PM	101	98	28	
	12 MN	99^8	88	22	
12/2/—	8 AM	97^2	64	12	BP 126/76
	4 PM	98^4	86	14	
12/3/—	8 AM	100	96	24	BP 114/76
	12 NOON	99^2	86	18	
	4 PM	99^8	88	22	
	8 PM	98^8	80	18	
12/4/—	8 AM	97^8	88	16	BP 118/78
	4 PM	98^6	80	18	
12/5/—	8 AM	97^2	68	14	BP 118/76
	4 PM	98^4	80	18	Discharged

GRAPHIC CHART

Family Name		First Name	Attending Physician			Room No.	Hosp. No.

Date									
Day in Hospital									
Day P O or P P									

	Hour	AM 4 8 12	PM 4 8 12	AM 4 8 12	PM 4 8 12	AM 4 8 12	PM 4 8 12	AM 4 8 12	PM 4 8 12	AM 4 8 12	PM 4 8 12	AM 4 8 12	PM 4 8 12	AM 4 8 12	PM 4 8 12
TEMPERATURE	106														
	105														
	104														
	103														
	102														
	101														
	100														
	99 Normal														
	98														
	97														
	96														
PULSE	150														
	140														
	130														
	120														
	110														
	100														
	90														
	80														
	70														
	60														
RESPIRATION	50														
	40														
	30														
	20														
	10														

Blood Pressure								
Fluid Intake								
Urine								
Defecation								
Weight								

ASSIGNMENT SHEET #5

Grade _____ Name _____

INTRODUCTION: On January 1, 20— Jim Johnson was admitted to Ram Hospital by Dr. Imhoff. The diagnosis was hepatitis and exhaustion from too much holiday celebration. Dr. Imhoff placed the patient in isolation. This assignment will allow you to perfect your skills on graphing TPRs.

INSTRUCTIONS: Record all of the following information on a blank graphic chart.

ROOM: 238   HOSPITAL NO.: 54-56-54   WEIGHT: 206 lb

Date	Time	T	P	R	Notes
1/1/——	12 NOON	103^4 R	136	38	BP 138/84
	4 PM	104^6 R	136	46	Aspirin Gr X
	8 PM	102^4 R	120	30	
	12 MN	103^2 R	130	36	Aspirin Gr XX
1/2/——	4 AM	100^4 R	116	24	
	8 AM	99^6 R	98	18	BP 124/78
	12 NOON	98^4	76	18	
	4 PM	99^6	94	24	
	8 PM	101^2	108	34	
	12 MN	103^8 R	120	42	Aspirin Gr X
1/3/——	4 AM	100^4 R	96	24	
	8 AM	99^6 R	84	18	BP 128/76
	12 NOON	99^8	88	22	
	4 PM	98^4	80	16	
	8 PM	98^8	86	18	
1/4/——	8 AM	97^2 Ax	68	12	BP 118/78
	12 NOON	98^4	76	18	
	4 PM	98^6	122	28	
	8 PM	99^4	86	18	
1/5/——	8 AM	97^6 Ax	62	14	BP 120/80
	4 PM	99^8	88	20	
	8 PM	102^6 R	94	28	Aspirin Gr XX
	12 PM	99^4 R	86	20	
1/6/——	8 AM	98^2	74	16	BP 124/72
	12 NOON	98^8	86	18	
	4 PM	98^8	90	18	
1/7/——	8 AM	97^4	64	12	BP 128/74
	8 PM	98^6	62	18	
1/8/——	8 AM	97^6	66	14	BP 120/68
	4 PM	98^4	82	12	

GRAPHIC CHART

Family Name		First Name	Attending Physician		Room No.	Hosp. No.

Date	
Day in Hospital	
Day P O or P P	

	Hour	A M	P M	A M	P M	A M	P M	A M	P M	A M	P M	A M	P M	A M	P M	A M	P M
		4 8 12	4 8 12	4 8 12	4 8 12	4 8 12	4 8 12	4 8 12	4 8 12	4 8 12	4 8 12	4 8 12	4 8 12	4 8 12	4 8 12	4 8 12	4 8 12

TEMPERATURE

106
105
104
103
102
101
100
99 Normal
98
97
96

PULSE

150
140
130
120
110
100
90
80
70
60

RESPIRATION

50
40
30
20
10

Blood Pressure	
Fluid Intake	
Urine	
Defecation	
Weight	

CHAPTER 13:6 MEASURING AND RECORDING APICAL PULSE

ASSIGNMENT SHEET

Grade _____ Name _____

INTRODUCTION: The following assignment will help you review the main facts regarding apical pulse.

INSTRUCTIONS: Read the information about Measuring and Recording an Apical Pulse. In the space provided, print the word(s) that best answers the question.

1. Define *apical pulse*.
   A pulse count taken c̄ a stethescope at the apex of the heart.

2. List two (2) diseases or conditions a patient may have that would require that an apical pulse be taken.
   - irregular heartbeats
   - hardening of the arteries

3. Why are apical pulses usually taken on infants and children?
   They have very rapid pulse counts.

4. What causes the lubb-dupp heart sounds that are heard while taking an apical pulse?
   The closing of the heart valves.

5. What should you do if you hear any abnormal sounds or beats while taking an apical pulse?
   Report the immediately to your supervisor.

6. What causes a pulse deficit or a higher rate for an apical pulse than a radial pulse?
   When the heart doesn't produce enough blood to create a pulse or when the heart beats too fast.

7. Calculate the pulse deficit for the following readings.

   Apical pulse 104, radial pulse 80: 24

   Apical pulse 142, radial pulse 96: 46

   Apical pulse 86, radial pulse 86: 0

8. How is the stethoscope cleaned before and after an apical pulse is taken?
   Using alcohol or a disenfectant wipe.

Name _____   Date _____

Evaluated by _____

DIRECTIONS: Practice measuring and recording an apical pulse according to the criteria listed. When you are ready for your final check, give this sheet to your instructor.

PROFICIENT

Measuring and Recording Apical Pulse	Points Possible	Peer Check Yes	Peer Check No	Final Check* Yes	Final Check* No	Points Earned**	Comments
1. Assembles equipment and supplies. Cleans earpieces and bell/diaphragm with disinfectant	5						
2. Washes hands	5						
3. Introduces self, identifies patient, and explains procedure	5						
4. Avoids unnecessary exposure of patient	6						
5. Places stethoscope in ears properly	7						
6. Places stethoscope on apical area	7						
7. Counts 1 full minute	7						
8. Obtains pulse count accurate to ± 2 beats per minute	15						
9. Notes rhythm and volume of pulse	10						
10. Records apical pulse information correctly	10						
11. Checks patient before leaving	6						
12. Cleans and replaces equipment	5						
13. Washes hands	5						
14. Recognizes an abnormal measurement and reports it immediately	7						
Totals	100						

*   Final Check: Instructor or authorized person evaluates.
** Points Earned: Points possible times each "yes" check.

CHAPTER 13:7 MEASURING AND RECORDING BLOOD PRESSURE

ASSIGNMENT SHEET #1

Grade _____ Name _____

INTRODUCTION: The following assignment will help you review the main facts regarding blood pressure.

INSTRUCTIONS: Read the information about Measuring and Recording Blood Pressure. Then answer the following questions in the spaces provided.

1. Define *blood pressure.*
   A measurement of the pressure that the blood exerts on the walls of the arteries

2. Define *systolic.*
   Occurs when the left ventricle is contracting.

3. Define *diastolic.*
   Constant pressure when the heart is at rest.

4. The average reading for systolic pressure is ___120 mmHg___ with a range of ___100-140 mmHg___

5. The average reading for diastolic pressure is ___80 mmHg___ with a range of ___60-90 mmHg___.

6. What is the pulse pressure if the blood pressure is 136/72?
   64 mmHg

7. Hypertension is indicated when pressures are greater than ___140___ systolic and ___90___ diastolic.

8. List three (3) causes of hypotension.
   - heart failure
   - dehydration
   - depression

9. What is orthostatic, or postural, hypotension? What causes it?
   Its when there is a sudden drop in both the systolic and diastolic pressures due to moving from lying to sitting/standing.

10. List three (3) factors that can increase blood pressure.
    - excitment
    - Stimulant drugs
    - smoking

11. List three (3) factors that can decrease or lower blood pressure.
   - sleep
   - depressant drugs
   - shock

12. Why does OSHA discourage the use of mercury sphygmomanometers?
   There is a possibility of a spill and contamination.

13. a. Record the following blood pressure readings correctly.

1	Systolic	128	Diastolic	92	36 128/92
2	Diastolic	84	Systolic	188	104 188/84
3	Systolic	136	Diastolic	76	60 136/76
4	Diastolic	118	Systolic	210	92 210/118

   b. Name all the above readings that fall within normal range.
   1, 3

   c. Name the above readings that do not fall within normal range.
   2, 4

14. Why is it important to use the correct size cuff?
   The wrong size will give inaccurate readings.

Med
Tech

ASSIGNMENT SHEET #2

Grade _____   Name _____

INTRODUCTION: The mercury gauge is a long column. Each mark represents 2 mm Hg. Complete this assignment sheet to learn how to record readings from this mercury gauge.

INSTRUCTIONS: In the space provided, place the reading to which the arrow is pointing.

1. 298
2. 288
3. 280
4. 274
5. 268
6. 258
7. 248
8. 242
9. 232
10. 226
11. 216
12. 210
13. 204
14. 192
15. 186
16. 176
17. 166
18. 160
19. 150
20. 146
21. 140
22. 132
23. 128
24. 120
25. 114
26. 106
27. 98
28. 94
29. 86
30. 74
31. 68
32. 60
33. 54
34. 48
35. 38

CHAPTER 13:7 READING AN ANEROID SPHYGMOMANOMETER

ASSIGNMENT SHEET #3

Grade _____ Name _____

INTRODUCTION: The aneroid gauge is a common gauge on many sphygmomanometers. Each line represents 2 mm Hg pressure. Complete this sheet to practice reading the gauge.

INSTRUCTIONS: In the spaces provided, place the reading to which the arrow is pointing.

1. _____20_____
2. _____34_____
3. _____42_____
4. _____52_____
5. _____62_____
6. _____76_____
7. _____82_____
8. _____90_____
9. _____98_____
10. _____104_____
11. _____116_____
12. _____130_____
13. _____134_____

14. _____142_____
15. _____150_____
16. _____158_____
17. _____170_____
18. _____178_____
19. _____186_____
20. _____198_____
21. _____208_____
22. _____222_____
23. _____236_____
24. _____244_____
25. _____260_____
26. _____276_____

Name _____ Date _____

Evaluated by _____

DIRECTIONS: Practice measuring and recording blood pressure according to the criteria listed. When you are ready for your final check, give this sheet to your instructor.

PROFICIENT

Measuring and Recording Blood Pressure	Points Possible	Peer Check Yes	No	Final Check* Yes	No	Points Earned**	Comments
1. Assembles equipment and supplies. Cleans stethoscope earpieces and bell/disk with a disinfectant	3						
2. Washes hands	3						
3. Introduces self and identifies patient	3						
4. Explains procedure	3						
5. Uses correct size cuff and applies it correctly	4						
6. Determines palpatory systolic pressure	4						
7. Deflates cuff and waits 30-60 seconds	4						
8. Places stethoscope in ears correctly	4						
9. Locates brachial artery	4						
10. Inflates cuff 30 mm Hg above palpatory systolic pressure	4						
11. Uses aneroid sphygmomanometer:							
Places gauge correctly	4						
Untangles tubing	4						
Reads pressure to ± 2 mm Hg	8						
Records correctly	4						
12. Uses mercury sphygmomanometer:							
Sets on flat surface	4						
Reads to ± 2 mm Hg	8						
Records correctly	4						
13. Reads adult diastolic as cessation of sound	5						
14. Reads child diastolic as change in sound	5						
15. Checks patient for comfort and safety	4						
16. Cleans stethoscope earpieces and bell/disk with a disinfectant	4						
17. Replaces equipment	3						
18. Washes hands	3						
19. Recognizes an abnormal measurement and reports it immediately	4						
Totals	100						

* Final Check: Instructor or authorized person evaluates.
** Points Earned: Points possible times each "yes" check.

ASSIGNMENT SHEET

Grade _____ Name _____

INTRODUCTION: The following assignment will help you review the main facts on general guidelines for first aid.

INSTRUCTIONS: Study the information on Providing First Aid. In the space provided, print the word(s) that best answers the question or completes the statement.

1. Define first aid.
   Immediate care that is given to the victim of an Injury or illness to minimize the effects of the injury or illness until experts can take over.

2. Using the correct first aid methods can mean the difference between ___*life*___ and ___*death*___, or ___*recovery*___ versus ___*permanent disability*___

3. The type of first aid treatment you provide will vary depending on several factors. List three (3) factors that may affect any action taken.
   1) enviornment   *3) equipment/supplies on hand*
   2) Others present   *4) availability of medical help*

4. Identify three (3) senses that can alert you to an emergency.
   1) unusual sounds (screams)   *3) breaking glass*
   2) calls for help   *4) screeching tires*

5. What action should you take if you notice that it is not safe to approach the scene of an accident?
   Call for professional help immediately.

6. What is the first thing you should determine when you get to the victim?
   Determine if the victim is conscious.

7. Why is it important to avoid moving a victim whenever possible?
   They can become more severely injured by being moved.

8. List five (5) kinds of information that should be reported while calling emergency medical services (EMS).
   1) Describe the situation   *4) phone number from which you're calling*
   2) actions taken
   3) exact location   *5) assistance required*
   6) number of people involved

9. What should you do if a person refuses to give consent for care?

Do not give care and have someone witness the person not giving their consent.

10. What is triage?

A method of prioritizing treatment.

11. Identify six (6) life-threatening emergencies that must be cared for first.

1) no breathing   4) persistent pain in chest
2) no pulse   5) vomiting / passing blood
3) severe bleeding   6) poisoning

12. List four (4) sources of information you can use to find out the details regarding an accident, injury, or illness.

1) victim   3) items at the scene
2) others present   4) bracelet, necklace,
                          medicine card

13. How can you reassure the victim?

Talk in a calm, confident voice.

14. Why shouldn't you discuss the victim's condition with observers at the scene?

The victim's right to privacy.

15. While providing first aid to the victim, make every attempt to avoid further **movement**. Provide only the treatment you are **certified** to provide.

CHAPTER 14:2 PERFORMING CARDIOPULMONARY RESUSCITATION (CPR)

ASSIGNMENT SHEET

Grade _____ Name _____

INTRODUCTION: This assignment will help you review the main facts regarding CPR.

INSTRUCTIONS: Review the information on Performing Cardiopulmonary Resuscitation (CPR). In the space provided, print the word(s) that best completes the statement or answers the question.

1. CPR stands for _Cardiopulmonary Resuscitation_.

2. What do the ABCDs of CPR represent?
   Airway
   Breathing
   Circulation
   Defibrilation

3. How does biological death differ from clinical death?
   - Clinical: occurs when the heart stops beating
   - Biological: the death of the body cells

4. When does biological death occur?
   4-6 minutes after clinical death

5. What two (2) methods can be used to open the airway?
   1) Place one hand on the victims forehead and the other under the chin and gently tilt the head back w/o closing the mouth.
   2) lift the chin w/o tilting the head back.

6. What is an AED? How is it used?
   - Automated External Defibrillaters
   - used to send an electronic shock to the heart to try to restore the normal pattern.

7. What should you determine first before starting CPR?
   - evaluate the victims condition

8. Identify each of the following situations as either a "call first" or "call fast" emergency.

   a. any victim of submersion or near-drowning: Call fast

   b. an unconscious adult or child 8 years old or older: Call first

   c. an unconscious infant with a high risk for heart problems: Call first

   d. an unconscious infant or child less than 8 years old: Call fast

   e. any victim with cardiac arrest caused by trauma or a drug overdose: Call fast

9. What is the three point evaluation that is used to check for breathing?
~~1) Open the airway~~ 2) listen for breathing through nose + mouth
1) look for chest movement
3) feel for movement of air

10. What pulse site is checked to determine if compression is necessary?
Carotid

11. Why is it important to place the heel of the hand one finger's width above the substernal notch before giving chest compressions?
To minimize injury

12. To perform a one-person rescue on an adult victim, give ___15___ compressions followed by ___2___ respirations. Compressions are given at the rate of ___100___ per minute. ___four___ 15:2 cycles should be completed every minute. Pressure should be applied straight down to compress the sternum about ___1½___ inches or ___2___ centimeters.

13. What is the ratio of compressions to ventilations when two people are giving CPR to an adult victim?
15:2

14. During a two-person rescue, how can the person giving breaths check the effectiveness of the compressions?
Check the carotid pulse

15. To rescue an infant, both the infant's _nose_ and the _mouth_ are covered for ventilations. Two fingers are placed on the sternum _1 finger width_ below a line drawn between the nipples, and the sternum is compressed _½ - 1_ inches or _1.3-2.5_ centimeters. Compressions are given at the rate of at least _100_ per minute. After each _5_ compressions, give one ventilation for a ratio of _5_ : _1_ compressions to ventilations.

16. CPR for a child is used when the child is under 8 years of age. Compressions are given at the rate of _100_ per minute. The heel of one hand is placed on the sternum _1 finger width_ above the _substernal notch_ The sternum is compressed _1 - 1½_ inches or _2.5-3.8_ centimeters. The ratio of compressions to ventilations is _5_ : _1_ .

17. What should you do for a choking victim who is conscious, coughing, and able to breathe?
Ecourage the victim to cough hard.

18. Briefly list the sequence of steps used to remove an obstruction in an unconscious adult victim who has an obstructed airway.
- 5 abdominal thrusts
- mouth sweep
- open the airway
- attempt to ventilate

19. Briefly list the sequence of steps used to remove an obstruction in an infant with an obstructed airway.

-5 back blows
-5 Chest thrusts
-Check the mouth
-fingersweep
-attempt to ventilate

20. You have tried to remove an obstruction from an airway for several minutes, but the airway is still blocked. Should you check the pulse and start chest compressions at this point? Why or why not?

No, there is no valve.

21. List six (6) reasons for stopping CPR once it is started.

1) victim recovers and starts to breathe
2) qualified help arrives & takes over
3) doctor orders you to discontinue
4) rescuer is physically exhausted
5) scene becomes unsafe
6) legal, valid DNR order

Name _____ Date _____

Evaluated by _____

DIRECTIONS: Practice performing CPR with a one-person rescue according to the criteria listed. When you are ready for your final check, give this sheet to your instructor.

Performing Cardiopulmonary Resuscitation: One-Person Rescue	Points Possible	Peer Check		Final Check*		Points Earned**	Comments
		Yes	No	Yes	No		
PROFICIENT							
1. Assembles equipment and supplies and places manikin on firm surface	1						
2. Checks consciousness:							
Shakes victim by tapping shoulder	3						
Asks "Are you OK?"	3						
3. If the victim is unconscious, follows "call first, call fast" priorities	5						
4. Opens airway with head tilt/chin lift method or jaw-thrust maneuver if victim has suspected neck/spine injury	5						
5. Looks, listens, and feels for respirations for 5 but not more than 10 seconds	5						
6. Gives 2 slow breaths until the chest rises gently	5						
7. Palpates carotid pulse for 5 but not more than10 seconds	5						
8. Administers chest compressions as follows:							
Locates correct hand position on sternum	5						
Places heel of hands on chest with fingers off of chest	5						
Positions shoulders above sternum to apply vertical force	5						
Keeps elbows straight	5						
Compresses $1\frac{1}{2}$ to 2 inches	5						
Gives 15 compressions at rate of 100 per minute	5						
Counts "one and, two and . . ."	5						
9. Gives two ventilations	5						
10. Repeats cycle of 15 compressions and 2 ventilations giving 4 cycles every minute	5						
11. Checks pulse and breathing for 5 but not more than 10 seconds after 4 cycles	5						
12. Resumes CPR by giving 2 breaths and then continues 15:2 cycle	5						
13. Continues CPR unless:							
Victim recovers	2						
Qualified help takes over	2						
Physician orders you to discontinue attempt	2						
Too physically exhausted	2						
Scene suddenly becomes unsafe	2						
Presented with a valid DNR order	2						
14. Cleans and replaces all equipment used	1						
Totals	100						

* Final Check: Instructor or authorized person evaluates.

** Points Earned: Points possible times each "yes" check.

Name _____ Date _____

Evaluated by _____

DIRECTIONS: Practice performing CPR with a two-person rescue according to the criteria listed. When you are ready for your final check, give this sheet to your instructor.

PROFICIENT

Performing Cardiopulmonary Resuscitation: Two-Person Rescue	Points Possible	Peer Check Yes	No	Final Check* Yes	No	Points Earned**	Comments
1. Assembles equipment and supplies and places manikin on firm surface	2						
2. First rescuer begins CPR:							
Shakes victim	3						
Asks "Are you OK?"	3						
Opens airway	3						
Looks, listens, and feels for breating for 5 but not more than 10 seconds	3						
Gives 2 slow breaths until the chest rises gently	3						
Checks carotid pulse for 5 but not more than 10 seconds	3						
If no pulse, locates correct position for hands	3						
Administers chest compressions at the rate of 100 per minute	3						
Gives 2 ventilations after each 15 compressions	3						
3. Second rescuer goes to obtain help	4						
4. When second rescuer returns, the first rescuer indicates "take over compressions"	4						
5. First rescuer completes 15:2 cycle	4						
6. First rescuer does 5 but not more than 10 second pulse and breathingcheck, states "No pulse. Continue CPR," and gives 2 gentle breaths	4						
7. If second rescuer takes over compressions:							
Second rescuer finds correct hand placement during pulse and breathing check	4						
Second rescuer gives compressions at rate of 100 per minute	3						
Counts "one and, two and, etc."	3						
Pauses slightly after 15 compressions	3						
First rescuer gives 2 breaths after each 15 compressions	3						
Rescuers continue with 15:2 cycle with slight pause for ventilation	4						

Performing Cardiopulmonary Resuscitation: Two-Person Rescue	Points Possible	Peer Check		Final Check*		Points Earned**	Comments
		Yes	No	Yes	No		
8. Rescuers switch positions as follows:							
Compressor gives clear signal to change positions	3						
Compressor completes cycle of 15 compressions	3						
Ventilator gives 2 ventilations after 15 compression	3						
Compressor moves to head							
Checks pulse and breathing for 5 but not more than 10 seconds	3						
Gives 2 gentle breaths	3						
Says "No pulse," continue CPR	3						
Ventilator moves to chest							
Locates correct hand placement for compressions	4						
After new ventilator gives 2 breaths, begins compressions at rate of 100 per minute	3						
Rescuers continue with 15:2 cycle with slight pause for ventilation	4						
9. Rescuers continue CPR until help arrives, victim recovers, doctor orders attempt discontinued, scene suddenly becomes unsafe, or presented with DNR order	4						
10. Cleans and replaces all equipment used	2						
Totals	100						

* Final Check: Instructor or authorized person evaluates.
** Points Earned: Points possible times each "yes" check.

Name _____   Date _____

Evaluated by _____

DIRECTIONS: Practice performing CPR on infants according to the criteria listed. When you are ready for your final check, give this sheet to your instructor.

PROFICIENT

Performing Cardiopulmonary Resuscitation: Infants	Points Possible	Peer Check		Final Check*		Points Earned**	Comments
		Yes	No	Yes	No		
1. Assembles equipment and supplies and places manikin on firm surface	2						
2. Shakes gently and calls to infant	5						
3. Calls aloud for help and follows "call first, call fast" priorities	5						
4. Opens airway but does not tilt head as far back as an adult	6						
5. Looks, listens, and feels for breathing for 5 but not more than 10 seconds	6						
6. Gives 2 slow breaths	5						
Covers mouth and nose	5						
Watches for chest to rise gently	5						
7. Checks brachial pulse on infants for 5 but not more than 10 seconds	6						
8. Administers compressions:							
Places 2 fingers one finger's width below an imaginary line drawn between the nipples	6						
Gives compressions at rate of 100 per minute	6						
Counts 1, 2, 3, 4, 5, breathe	6						
Compresses $\frac{1}{2}$ to 1 inch or 1.4 to 2.5 centimeters	6						
Supports back or places victim on firm surface	6						
9. Gives one ventilation after every 5 compressions	6						
10. Repeats cycle of 5:1 with slight pause for ventilation	6						
11. Checks breathing and pulse after 1 minute—checks for 5 but not more than 10 seconds	6						
12. Continues CPR if no breathing or pulse by starting with one breath	5						
13. Cleans and replaces all equipment	2						
Totals	100						

* Final Check: Instructor or authorized person evaluates.
** Points Earned: Points possible times each "yes" check.

Name _____ Date _____

Evaluated by _____

DIRECTIONS: Practice performing CPR on children according to the criteria listed. When you are ready for your final check, give this sheet to your instructor.

PROFICIENT

Performing Cardiopulmonary Resuscitation: Children	Points Possible	Peer Check Yes	No	Final Check* Yes	No	Points Earned**	Comments
1. Assembles equipment and supplies and places manikin on firm surface	2						
2. Shakes gently and calls to child	5						
3. Obtains medical help as soon as possible following "call first, call fast" priorities	5						
4. Opens airway correctly	6						
5. Looks, listens, and feels for breathing for 5 but not more than 10 seconds	6						
6. Gives 2 slow breaths	5						
Covers nose and mouth or just mouth	5						
Watches for chest to rise	5						
7. Checks carotid pulse for 5 but not more than 10 seconds	6						
8. Administers compressions if no pulse:							
Places heel of one hand one finger's width above substernal notch	6						
Gives compressions at rate of 100 per minute	6						
Counts 1 and 2 and 3 and 4 and 5	6						
Compresses 1–1½ inches or 2.5 to 3.8 centimeters	6						
Supports back or places child on flat surface	6						
9. Gives 1 ventilation after every 5 compressions	6						
10. Repeats cycle of 5:1 with slight pause for ventilations	6						
11. Checks breathing and pulse for 5 but not more than 10 seconds after 1 minute	6						
12. Continues CPR if no breathing or pulse by starting with 1 breath	5						
13. Cleans and replaces all equipment	2						
Totals	100						

* Final Check: Instructor or authorized person evaluates.
** Points Earned: Points possible times each "yes" check.

Name _____   Date _____

Evaluated by _____

DIRECTIONS: Practice performing CPR on a conscious victim with an obstructed airway according to the criteria listed. When you are ready for your final check, give this sheet to your instructor. NOTE: Use only a manikin to perform thrusts.

PROFICIENT

Performing Cardiopulmonary Resuscitation: Obstructed Airway on Conscious Victim	Points Possible	Peer Check		Final Check*		Points Earned**	Comments
		Yes	No	Yes	No		
1. Assembles equipment and supplies and places manikin in upright position	5						
2. Determines if victim has an airway obstruction:							
Asks " Are you choking?"	5						
Checks if victim can cough, talk, or breathe	5						
3. Calls out for help	6						
4. Performs abdominal thrusts:							
Stands behind victim	8						
Wraps arms around victim's waist	8						
Places thumb side of fist above umbilicus but below xiphoid	8						
Grasps fist with other hand	8						
Uses quick upward thrusts	8						
5. Demonstrates chest thrusts for very obese or pregnant victim:							
Stands behind victim	4						
Wraps arms under victim's axillae	4						
Places thumb side of fist against center of sternum but well above xiphoid	4						
Grasps fist with other hand	4						
Thrusts inward	4						
6. Repeats thrusts until object expelled or victim loses consciousness	8						
7. Obtains medical help as soon as possible	6						
8. Replaces all equipment	5						
Totals	100						

* Final Check: Instructor or authorized person evaluates.
** Points Earned: Points possible times each "yes" check.

Name _____ Date _____

Evaluated by _____

DIRECTIONS: Practice performing CPR on an unconscious victim with an obstructed airway according to the criteria listed. When you are ready for your final check, give this sheet to your instructor.

PROFICIENT

Performing Cardiopulmonary Resuscitation: Obstructed Airway on Unconscious Victim	Points Possible	Peer Check Yes	No	Final Check* Yes	No	Points Earned**	Comments
1. Assembles equipment and supplies and places manikin on firm surface	1						
2. Shakes victim and asks "Are you OK?"	4						
3. If the victim is unconscious, follows "call first, call fast" priorities to call for medical help	4						
4. Opens airway with head tilt/chin lift method	4						
5. Looks, listens, and feels for breathing for 5 but not more than 10 seconds	4						
6. Attempts to give breaths	4						
7. When chest does not rise, repositions head and attempts to ventilate	4						
8. Gives abdominal thrusts as follows:							
Positions victim on back	4						
Straddles victim's thighs	4						
Places heel of one hand on abdomen above umbilicus but below xiphoid	4						
Places other hand on top of first hand	4						
Gives quick upward thrusts into the abdomen	5						
Gives 5 thrusts	5						
9. Checks for object in mouth as follows:							
Opens mouth by lifting lower jaw with thumb and fingers	4						
Uses index finger to sweep mouth with C-shape or hooking motion	4						
Removes object if visible	4						
10. Opens airway and attempts to ventilate	4						
11. If chest rises, continues with steps of CPR by checking carotid pulse	4						
12. If the chest does not rise, repositions head and attempts to ventilate	4						
13. If chest still does not rise, repeats cycle of 5 thrusts, mouth check, attempt to ventilate	4						

14:2F (cont.)

Performing Cardiopulmonary Resuscitation: Obstructed Airway on Unconscious Victim	Points Possible	Peer Check Yes	No	Final Check* Yes	No	Points Earned**	Comments
14. Continues repeating cycle until object removed and airway open or help comes	4						
15. Follows same sequence for infants but observes following variations:							
Gives 5 back blows by positioning infant face down with head lower than chest	4						
Gives 5 chest thrusts using 2 to 3 fingers one finger's width below an imaginary line drawn between nipples with infant positioned face up and head lower than chest	4						
Looks in mouth for object but sweeps mouth with finger only if object is seen	4						
Attempts to ventilate	4						
16. Cleans and replaces all equipment	1						
Totals	100						

* Final Check: Instructor or authorized person evaluates.
** Points Earned: Points possible times each "yes" check.

CHAPTER 14:3 PROVIDING FIRST AID FOR BLEEDING AND WOUNDS

ASSIGNMENT SHEET

Grade _____   Name _____

INTRODUCTION: This assignment will help you review the main facts about providing first aid for bleeding and wounds.

INSTRUCTIONS: Read the information on Providing First Aid for Bleeding and Wounds. In the space provided, print the word(s) that best completes the statement or answers the question.

1. What is the difference between a closed wound and an open wound?
   open - break in the skin or mucous membrane
   closed - no break in the skin or mucous membrane but injury occurs to the underlying tissue

2. First aid care for wounds must be directed at controlling _bleeding_ and preventing _infection_.

3. List the correct name for each of the following types of open wounds.

   a. Scrape on the skin: abrasion

   b. Cut or injury by sharp object: incision

   c. Jagged irregular injury with tearing: laceration

   d. Wound caused by sharp pointed object: puncture

   e. Tissue torn or separated from body: avulsion

   f. Body part cut off: amputation

4. Briefly describe the characteristics or signs and symptoms for each of the following types of bleeding.
   a. Arterial blood: abrasion spurts from a wound, heavy blood loss

   b. Venous blood: slow, steady, dark red

   c. Capillary blood: oozes, slowly, clots easily

5. List the four (4) methods for controlling bleeding in the order in which they should be used.
   1) direct pressure   3) pressure bandage
   2) elevation   4) pressure points

6. Name two (2) items that can be used to form a protective barrier while controlling bleeding.
   1) gloves
   2) plastic wrap

7. The main pressure point for the arm is the _brachial artery_
   The main pressure point in the leg is the _femoral artery_.

8. List four (4) ways to prevent infection while caring for minor wounds without severe bleeding.

1) wash your hands   3) use soap, water, + sterile gauze

2) wear gloves   4) wipe in an outward direction (away from the wound)

9. List five (5) signs of infection.

1) swelling
2) heat
3) redness
4) pain
5) fever

10. If a tetanus infection is a possibility, what first aid is necessary?

— find out when the persons last tetnus shot was

— get medical advice on the situation

11. How should objects embedded deep in the tissues be removed?

— they should be left in a let a physician take them out

12. List six (6) signs and symptoms of a closed wound.

1) pain   4) deformity

2) tenderness   5) cold / clammy skin

3) swelling   6) rapid / weak pulse

13. List four (4) first aid treatments for a victim of a closed wound.

1) check breathing   3) avoid unecessary movement

2) treat for shock   4) avoid giving fluids/food

14. What other condition must you be prepared to treat while caring for wounds?

— shock

15. At all times, remain __calm__ while providing first aid. Obtain _professional_ care as soon as possible.

Name _____   Date _____

Evaluated by _____

DIRECTIONS: Practice providing first aid for bleeding and wounds according to the criteria listed. When you are ready for your final check, give this sheet to your instructor.

Providing First Aid for Bleeding and Wounds	Points Possible	Peer Check Yes	Peer Check No	Final Check* Yes	Final Check* No	Points Earned**	Comments
1. Follows priority of care:							
Checks the scene	3						
Checks consciousness and breathing	3						
Calls emergency medical services	3						
Cares for victim	3						
2. Controls severe bleeding with direct pressure:							
Put on gloves or uses protective barrier	3						
Uses dressing over wound	3						
Applies pressure directly to wound	3						
Avoids releasing pressure to check bleeding	3						
Applies second dressing if first soaks through	3						
3. Elevates injured part while applying pressure if no fracture is present	5						
4. Applies pressure bandage to hold dressing in place:							
Maintains direct pressure and elevation	3						
Applies additional dressings over dressings on wound	3						
Secures dressings by wrapping with roller bandage in overlapping turns	3						
Ties off bandage with tie over dressings	3						
Checks pulse site below bandage	3						
Loosens and replaces bandage if signs of impaired circulation are present	3						
5. Applies pressure to pressure point if bleeding does not stop:							
Continues with direct pressure and elevation	4						
Applies pressure correctly to brachial artery in arm	4						
Applies pressure correctly to femoral artery in leg	4						
Releases pressure slowly when bleeding stops but continues with direct pressure and elevation	4						

PROFICIENT

14:3 (cont).

Providing First Aid for Bleeding and Wounds	Points Possible	Peer Check Yes	No	Final Check* Yes	No	Points Earned**	Comments
6. Removes gloves and washes hands thoroughly	4						
7. Observes for signs of shock and treats as necessary	4						
8. Reassures victim during care and remains calm	3						
9. Treats minor wounds without severe bleeding:							
Washes hands	2						
Puts on gloves	2						
Washes wound with soap, water and sterile gauze in outward motion	2						
Discards gauze after each use	2						
Rinses wound with cool water	2						
Blots dry with sterile gauze	2						
Applies sterile dressing	2						
Cautions victim to watch for signs of infection and get medical help	2						
Refers to doctor if danger of tetanus present	2						
Removes gloves and washes hands thoroughly	2						
10. Obtains medical help as soon as possible when needed for victim	3						
Totals	100						

* Final Check: Instructor or authorized person evaluates.
** Points Earned: Points possible times each "yes" check.

CHAPTER 14:4 PROVIDING FIRST AID FOR SHOCK

ASSIGNMENT SHEET

Grade _____ Name _____

INTRODUCTION: This assignment will help you review the main facts regarding shock.

INSTRUCTIONS: Review the information on Providing First Aid for Shock. In the space provided, print the word(s) that best completes the statement or answers the question.

1. Define *shock*.
   - *a clinical set of signs and symptoms associated w/ an inadequate supply of blood to body organs*

2. Name the two (2) main body organs affected by an inadequate supply of blood.
   1) brain
   2) heart

3. List six (6) causes of shock.
   1) hemorrhage   3) infection   5) stroke
   2) excessive pain   4) heart attack   (6) poisioning

4. Identify each of the following types of shock:

   a. caused by an acute infection: *septic*

   b. heat can not pump effectively because heart muscle is damaged: *cardiogenic*

   c. sever bleeding leads to a decrease in blood volume: *hemorrhagic*

   d. hypersensitive or allergic reaction causes body to release histamine: *anaphylactic*

   e. emotional distress causes sudden dilation of blood vessels: *psychogenic*

   f. loss of body fluid causes disruption in normal acid–base balance of body: *metabolic*

5. List ten (10) signs or symptoms of shock.
   1) pale/bluish skin   4) pulse rapid/weak   7) weakness   10) blurred
   2) cool skin   5) respirations rapid/shallow 8) anxiety   vision
   3) excessive perspiration 6) B/P low   9) thirst/nausea

6. Treatment for shock is directed at eliminating the *cause of shock*, improving *circulation*, providing *an adequate O₂ supply*, and maintaining *body temperature*.

7. The position for treating shock is based on the victim's injuries. Briefly list the best position for each of the following cases:

   a. Victim with neck or spine injuries: *don't move*

   b. Victim vomiting or bleeding from the mouth: *on the side*

   c. Victim with respiratory distress: *raise the head and shoulders*

   d. Position if none of the previous conditions is present: *on the back*

8. A shock victim at an accident scene has been covered with blankets. You notice the victim is perspiring. What should you do?
   Remove some of the blankets.

Name _____ Date _____

Evaluated by _____

DIRECTIONS: Practice providing first aid for shock according to the criteria listed. When you are ready for your final check, give this sheet to your instructor.

PROFICIENT

Providing First Aid for Shock	Points Possible	Peer Check Yes	No	Final Check* Yes	No	Points Earned**	Comments
1. Follows priorities:							
Checks the scene	4						
Checks consciousness and breathing	4						
Calls emergency medical services	4						
Cares for victim	4						
Controls bleeding	4						
2. Observes victim for signs of shock:							
Pale or bluish color to skin	2						
Cool, moist or clammy skin	2						
Diaphoresis	2						
Rapid, weak, irregular pulse	2						
Rapid, weak, irregular, shallow or labored respirations	2						
Low blood pressure	2						
Signs of weakness, apathy and/or confusion	2						
Nausea and/or vomiting	2						
Excessive thirst	2						
Restless or anxious	2						
Blurred vision	2						
Eyes sunken; vacant, dilated pupils	2						
3. Attempts to reduce shock by treating bleeding, providing oxygen, easing pain, and giving emotional support	6						
4. Positions victim according to injuries or illness:							
Avoids movement if neck or spine injury present	5						
Positions on side if vomiting or has a jaw/mouth injury	5						
Positions lying flat with head raised if victim having difficulty breathing	5						
Positions lying flat or with head raised slightly if head injury present	5						
Positions lying flat with feet raised 12 inches if none of the above conditions present	5						

Providing First Aid for Shock	Points Possible	Peer Check		Final Check*		Points Earned**	Comments
		Yes	No	Yes	No		
5. Places enough blankets on/under victim to prevent chilling but avoids overheating	5						
6. Avoids giving fluids by mouth if medical help is available, victim unconscious or convulsing, brain or abdominal injury, surgery possible, or nausea and vomiting noted	5						
7. Remains calm and reassures victim	5						
8. Observes and cares for victim until medical help obtained	6						
9. Replaces all equipment used	2						
10. Washes hands	2						
Totals	100						

* Final Check: Instructor or authorized person evaluates.
** Points Earned: Points possible times each "yes" check.

CHAPTER 14:5 PROVIDING FIRST AID
FOR POISONING

ASSIGNMENT SHEET

Grade _____   Name _____

INTRODUCTION: This assignment will help you review the main facts on providing first aid for poisoning.

INSTRUCTIONS: Read the information on Providing First Aid for Poisoning. In the space provided, print the word(s) that best completes the statement or answers the question.

1. List four (4) ways that poisoning can be caused.
   1) swallowing various substances   3) injecting substances
   2) inhaling poisonous gases   4) contacting the skin with poison

2. Treatment for poisoning will vary depending on the _____ type _____ of poison, the _____ injury _____ involved, and the method of _____ contact _____.

3. What is the first thing to do when a victim swallows a poison?
   Call poison control / physician immediately.

4. List three (3) types of information that should be given to a poison control center or physician.
   1) the substance taken   3) the time taken
   2) how much taken

5. What should you do if a conscious poison victim vomits?
   Place them on their side with their head slightly downward.

6. How should you position an unconscious poisoning victim who is breathing? Why?
   Place them on their side so the poison can drain out of their mouth.

7. List two (2) ways to induce vomiting.
   1) syrup of ipecac
   2) warm salt water

8. Why is activated charcoal used after a poisoning victim vomits?
   To help absorb any remaining poison.

9. List four (4) types of poison victims in whom vomiting should not be induced.
   1) unconscious victims   3) swallowed petroleum
   2) swallowed acid/alkali   4) burns on the lips/mouth

10. What is the first step of treatment for a victim who has been poisoned by inhaling gas?
    The victim must be removed from the area

11. How do you treat victims poisoned by chemicals splashing on the skin?
    Use water to wash the skin for at least 18-20 minutes.

12. List five (5) signs of an allergic reaction to an injected poison.
    1) skin hives
    2) bronchiole constriction
    3) narrow alveoli passages
    4) hypotension
    5) edema

Name _____ Date _____

Evaluated by _____

DIRECTIONS: Practice providing first aid for poisoning according to the criteria listed. When you are ready for your final check, give this sheet to your instructor.

PROFICIENT

Providing First Aid for Poisoning	Points Possible	Peer Check Yes	No	Final Check* Yes	No	Points Earned**	Comments
1. Follows steps of priority care:							
Checks the scene	2						
Checks consciousness and breathing	2						
Calls emergency medical services	2						
Cares for victim	2						
Controls bleeding	2						
2. Checks victim for signs of poisoning by noting the following points:							
Burns on lips or mouth	2						
Odor	2						
Presence of poison container	2						
Presence of substance on victim or in mouth	2						
Information obtained from victim or observers	2						
3. Provides first aid for conscious victim who has swallowed poison:							
Determines type poison, how much taken, and when	2						
Calls poison control center or physician	2						
Follows instructions from poison control center	2						
Saves sample of any vomited material	2						
4. Induces vomiting only if told to do so, no medical help available, and *none* of the following present:							
Victim unconscious	2						
Victim convulsing	2						
Burns on lips or mouth	2						
Victim ingested acid, alkali, or petroleum product	2						
5. Provides first aid for unconscious victim:							
Checks breathing and gives artificial respiration if needed	3						
Positions breathing victim on side	3						
Calls poison control center and obtains medical help	3						

14:5 (cont.)

Providing First Aid for Poisoning	Points Possible	Peer Check		Final Check*		Points Earned**	Comments
		Yes	No	Yes	No		
Saves any vomitus and container with poison	3						
6. Provides first aid for a victim with chemicals or poisons splashed on the skin as follows:							
Washes area with large amounts of water	2						
Removes clothing containing substance	2						
Obtains medical help for burns/injuries	2						
7. Provides first aid for a victim who has come in contact with poisonous plants as follows:							
Washes area with soap and water	2						
Removes contaminated clothing	2						
Applies lotions or baking soda paste	2						
Obtains medical help if condition severe	2						
8. Provides first aid for victim who has inhaled poisonous gas as follows:							
Takes deep breath before entering area	2						
Holds breath while removing victim from area	2						
Checks breathing and gives artificial respiration as needed	2						
Obtains medical help	2						
9. Provides first aid for victim with insect bite/sting or snakebite:							
Positions affected area below level of heart	2						
Treats insect bite/sting:							
Removes embedded stinger by scraping stinger away from skin with the edge of a rigid card	2						
Washes area with soap and water	2						
Applies sterile dressing	2						
Applies cold pack	2						
Treats snakebite:							
Washes wound	2						
Immobilizes injured area	2						
Monitors breathing and gives artificial respiration if necessary	2						
Obtains medical help	2						
Watches for signs/symptoms of allergic reaction	3						
10. Observes all victims for signs of shock and treats as necessary	3						
11. Reassures victim while providing care	3						
12. Obtains medical help for any victim as soon as possible	3						
Totals	100						

* Final Check: Instructor or authorized person evaluates.
** Points Earned: Points possible times each "yes" check.

CHAPTER 14:6 PROVIDING FIRST AID FOR BURNS

ASSIGNMENT SHEET

Grade _____ Name _____

INTRODUCTION: This sheet will help you review the main facts on burns and first aid treatment for burns.

INSTRUCTIONS: Review the information on Providing First Aid for Burns. In the space provided, print the word(s) that best completes the statement or answers the question.

1. Define *burn*.
   An injury that can be caused by fire, heat, chemical agents, radiation, and/or electricity.

2. Briefly list the characteristics or signs and symptoms for each of the following types of burns:

First degree or superficial	Second degree or partial-thickness	Third degree or full-thickness
- top layer of skin - heals 5-6 days - reddend/discolored skin - mild swelling/pain	- top layers of the skin - blister/vessicle forms - red, mottled skin - swelling - skin surface appears wet - painful - 3-4 weeks healing	- all layers of skin + underlying tissue - white/charred apperance - painful/painless - life threatening

3. First aid treatment for burns is directed at removing _sources of heat_, cooling _affected skin_, covering _burn_, relieving _pain_, observing and treating _for shock_, and preventing _infection_.

4. Identify five (5) times when medical care should be obtained for burn victims.
   1) if more than 15% body burned   3) victim has difficulty breathing
   2) burns affect face/respiratory tract   4) burns cover more than 1 part of the body
   5) burns resulted from chemicals

5. What is the main treatment for superficial and mild, partial-thickness burns?
   Cool the area by flushing it with water.

6. Why is a sterile dressing applied to a burn?
   To prevent infection.

7. If blisters appear on a burn, how should you treat these?
   Don't burst them because this will cause infection.

8. How should severe second degree or third-degree burns be treated?
   They should be treated professionally.

9. If chemicals or irritating gases burn the eyes, how should the eyes be treated?
   Flush the eyes with large amounts of water until medical help arrives.

10. Why is shock frequently noted in victims with severe burns?
    Loss of body fluids can occur quickly.

Name _____ Date _____

Evaluated by _____

DIRECTIONS: Practice providing first aid for burns according to the criteria listed. When you are ready for your final check, give this sheet to your instructor.

PROFICIENT

Providing First Aid for Burns	Points Possible	Peer Check Yes	No	Final Check* Yes	No	Points Earned**	Comments
1. Follows priorities:							
Checks the scene	2						
Checks consciousness and breathing	2						
Calls emergency medical services	2						
Cares for victim	2						
Controls bleeding	2						
2. Identifies type of burn present as follows:							
First degree or superficial: reddened	3						
Second degree or partial-thickness: red, wet, painful, swollen, blister	3						
Third degree or full-thickness: white or charred with destruction of tissue	3						
3. Provides first aid for superficial or mild partial-thickness burns:							
Cools burn by flushing it with large amounts of cool water	3						
Blots dry gently with sterile gauze	3						
Applies dry sterile dressing	3						
Avoids breaking blisters	3						
Elevates burned area if possible	3						
Obtains medical help if necessary	3						
4. Provides first aid for severe partial-thickness or all full-thickness burns:							
Obtains medical help immediately	3						
Applies dry sterile dressing	3						
Avoids removing charred clothing from area	3						
Elevates hands and arms or legs and feet if affected	3						
Elevates head if victim in respiratory distress	3						
5. Provides first aid for chemical burns as follows:							
Flushes area with large amounts of water	3						
Removes contaminated clothing	3						
Continues flushing with large amounts of cool water	3						
Obtains medical help	3						

Providing First Aid for Burns	Points Possible	Peer Check		Final Check*		Points Earned**	Comments
		Yes	No	Yes	No		
6. Provides first aid for burns of the eye as follows:							
Asks victim to remove glasses or contacts	2						
Positions victim with head to side and injured eye down	3						
Pours water from inner to outer part of eye	3						
Irrigates for 15–30 minutes or until medical help arrives	3						
Obtains medical help	3						
7. Observes for signs of shock in all victims and treats as necessary	3						
8. Reassures victim and remains calm	3						
9. Obtains medical help for any of the following:							
Burns extensive (Over 15% of surface of adult body, 10% in child)	2						
Third-degree or full-thickness burns	2						
Victim under 5 or over 60 with partial-thickness burn	2						
Burns of the face	2						
Signs of shock	2						
Respiratory distress	2						
Burns of the eye/eyes	2						
Chemical burns on the skin	2						
Totals	100						

* Final Check: Instructor or authorized person evaluates.
** Points Earned: Points possible times each "yes" check.

CHAPTER 14:7 PROVIDING FIRST AID FOR HEAT EXPOSURE

ASSIGNMENT SHEET

Grade _____ Name _____

INTRODUCTION: This assignment will help you review the main facts regarding conditions caused by exposure to heat.

INSTRUCTIONS: Review the information on Providing First Aid for Heat Exposure. In the space provided, print the word(s) that best completes the statement or answers the question.

1. What occurs when the body is over exposed to heat?
   It may cause a chemical imbalance in the body which may eventually lead to death.

2. What are heat cramps?
   Muscle pains and spasms that result from the loss of water and salt through perspiration.

3. List three (3) first aid treatments for heat cramps.
   1) firm pressure applied to the muscle   3) small sips of water or rehydration drinks
   2) resting in a cool area

4. List six (6) signs or symptoms of heat exhaustion.
   1) pale/clammy skin   4) weakness
   2) profuse perspiration   5) headache
   3) fatigue/tiredness   6) muscle cramps

5. List three (3) first aid treatments for heat exhaustion.
   1) moving the victim to a cooler area
   2) loosening/removing excess clothing
   3) applying cool, wet cloths

6. How does internal body temperature differ in heat exhaustion and heat stroke?
   exhaustion – rises externally
   stroke – rises internally

7. List three (3) signs and symptoms of heat stroke.
   1) red, hot, dry skin
   2) rapid, strong pulse
   3) high body temperature

8. High body temperatures (such as 105° F or 41°C) can cause ___convulsions___ and/or ___death___ in a very short period of time.

9. List three (3) first aid treatments for heat stroke.
   1) placed in a tub of cool water
   2) sponged w/ cool water
   3) ice packs

10. Identify two (2) precautions a victim should take after recovering from any condition caused by exposure to heat.
    1) avoid abnormally hot temperatures for several days
    2) drink sufficient amounts of water / eat salts

Name _____ Date _____

Evaluated by _____

DIRECTIONS: Practice providing first aid for heat exposure according to the criteria listed. When you are ready for your final check, give this sheet to your instructor.

PROFICIENT

Providing First Aid for Heat Exposure	Points Possible	Peer Check Yes	No	Final Check* Yes	No	Points Earned**	Comments
1. Follows priorities:							
Checks the scene	2						
Checks consciousness and breathing	2						
Calls emergency medical services	2						
Cares for victim	2						
Controls bleeding	2						
2. Observes signs to determine condition as follows:							
Heat cramps: muscle pain or spasm	3						
Heat exhaustion: close to normal body temperature, skin pale and clammy, diaphoresis, nausea, headache, weakness, dizziness, fatigue	4						
Heat stroke: high body temperature; skin hot, red and dry; weak or unconscious	4						
3. Provides first aid for heat cramps:							
Applies firm pressure to muscle with hand	4						
Lies victim down in cool area	4						
Gives victim small sips of cool water to total 4 ounces in 15 minutes	4						
Obtains medical help if cramps continue	4						
4. Provides first aid for heat exhaustion:							
Moves to cool area	3						
Positions lying down with feet elevated 12 inches	3						
Loosens tight clothing	3						
Applies cool wet cloths	3						
Gives victim small sips of cool water to total 4 ounces in 15 minutes	3						
Discontinues water if victim complains of nausea and/or vomits	3						
Obtains medical help if necessary	3						

14:7 (cont.)

Providing First Aid for Heat Exposure	Points Possible	Peer Check		Final Check*		Points Earned**	Comments
		Yes	No	Yes	No		
5. Provides first aid for heat stroke as follows:							
Moves to cool area	4						
Removes excess clothing	4						
Sponges skin with cool water; places ice or cold packs on victim's wrists, ankles, and in axillary or groin areas; or puts victim in tub of cool water	4						
Positions victim on side if vomiting occurs	4						
Obtains medical help immediately	4						
6. Observes for sign of shock and treats for shock in all victims	5						
7. Reassures victim while providing care, remains calm	5						
8. Obtains medical help for any of the following victims:							
Heat cramps do not subside	4						
Heat exhaustion victim with vomiting or shock	4						
All heat stroke victims	4						
Totals	100						

*   Final Check: Instructor or authorized person evaluates.
** Points Earned: Points possible times each "yes" check.

CHAPTER 14:8 PROVIDING FIRST AID FOR COLD EXPOSURE

ASSIGNMENT SHEET

Grade _____ Name _____

INTRODUCTION: This assignment will help you review the main facts on first aid for cold exposure.

INSTRUCTIONS: Read the information on Providing First Aid for Cold Exposure. In the space provided, prin the word(s) that best completes the statement or answers the question.

1. List three (3) factors that affect the degree of injury caused by exposure to the cold.
   1) wind velocity
   2) amount of humidity
   3) length of exposure

2. List five (5) symptoms that can result from prolonged exposure to the cold.
   1) shivering   4) low body temperature
   2) numbness   5) poor cordination
   3) weakhness/
      drowsiness

3. List three (3) first aid treatments for hypothermia.
   1) Get the victim to a warm area
   2) remove wet clothing
   3) warm the victim

4. What is frostbite?
   The freezing of tissue fluids accompanied by damage to the skin and underlying tissues.

5. List four (4) symptoms of frostbite.
   1) redness+tingling   3) white or greysh-yellow color
   2) pale, glossy skin   4) blisters

6. Name four (4) common sites for frostbite.
   1) fingers/toes   3) nose
   2) ears   4) cheeks

7. What temperature water should be used to warm a body part injured by frostbite?
   100-104°F

8. Why is it important not to rub or massage a body part affected by frostbite?
   It could cause gangrene

9. How should you treat blisters that form on frost-damaged skin?
   Don't burst or open them.

10. Why do you place sterile gauze between fingers or toes that have been injured by frostbite?
    To prevent rubbing and causing further injury.

Name _____ Date _____

Evaluated by _____

DIRECTIONS: Practice providing first aid for cold exposure according to the criteria listed. When you are ready for your final check, give this sheet to your instructor.

PROFICIENT

Providing First Aid for Cold Exposure	Points Possible	Peer Check Yes	No	Final Check* Yes	No	Points Earned**	Comments
1. Follows priorities:							
Checks the scene	3						
Checks consciousness and breathing	3						
Calls emergency medical services	3						
Cares for victim	3						
Controls severe bleeding	3						
2. Observes for signs of exposure to cold	7						
3. Checks skin for signs of frostbite	6						
4. Moves victim to warm area	6						
5. Removes wet or frozen clothing and loosens constrictive clothing	6						
6. Warms victim slowly by wrapping in blankets or putting on dry clothing	6						
7. Immerses frostbitten part in water at 100°–104° F (37.8°–40° C)	6						
8. Discontinues warming when skin flushed	6						
9. Dries area or body by blotting gently	6						
10. Places sterile gauze between fingers and toes affected by frostbite	6						
11. Positions victim lying down with affected parts elevated	6						
12. Observes and treats for shock	6						
13. Gives warm liquids to victim if victim conscious and not nauseated or vomiting	6						
14. Reassures victim while providing care	6						
15. Obtains medical help as soon as possible	6						
Totals	100						

* Final Check: Instructor or authorized person evaluates.
** Points Earned: Points possible times each "yes" check.

CHAPTER 14:9 PROVIDING FIRST AID FOR BONE AND JOINT INJURIES

ASSIGNMENT SHEET

Grade _____ Name _____

INTRODUCTION: This assignment will help you review the main facts regarding bone and joint injuries.

INSTRUCTIONS: Read the information on Providing First Aid for Bone and Joint Injuries. In the space provided, print the word(s) that best completes the statement or answers the question.

1. Define each of the following:

   fracture: a break in a bone

   dislocation: the end of a bone is displaced from a joint or moved from normal p

   sprain: injury to a tissue surrounding a joint

   strain: the overstretching of a muscle

2. What is the difference between a closed or simple fracture and an open or compound fracture?

   1) Closed/Simple - bone break not accompanied by an external/open wound

   2) Open/Compound - bone break accompanied by an external/open wound on the skin

3. List six (6) signs and symptoms of a fracture.

   1) deformity   4) swelling + discoloration
   2) limited/loss of motion   5) discoloration
   3) pain + tenderness   6) protrusion of a bone

4. Treatment for fractures is directed at maintaining ___respirations___, treating ___shock___, keeping the broken bone from ___moving___, and preventing further ___injury___.

5. List four (4) signs and symptoms of a dislocation.

   1) deformity   3) swelling
   2) limited/abnormal movement   4) discoloration

6. Why is movement of the injured part dangerous when a dislocation has occurred?

   Movement can lead to additional injuries to nerves, blood vessels, and other tissues.

7. List four (4) signs and symptoms of a sprain.

   1) swelling   3) discoloration
   2) pain   4) impaired motion

8. List three (3) first aid treatments for a sprain.

   1) application of cold to decrease pain and swelling
   2) elevation of the effected part
   3) rest

9. Why are cold applications used to treat a sprain or strain?

    To decrease swelling and pain.

    Why are warm applications used to treat a strain?

    Warmth relaxes the muscles.

10. List six (6) different types of materials that can be used for splints.

    1) Cardboard   4) pillows
    2) newspapers   5) boards
    3) blankets   6) padded boards

11. List three (3) basic principles that should be followed when splints are applied.

    1) Splints should be long enough to immobilize the joint above + below the injured area

    2) Splints should be padded

    3) Splints must be applied so that they don't put pressure directly over the site of injury

12. How can you test that an air splint is inflated properly?

    Use your thumb to slightly apply pressure. If inflated right a small indentation will be there.

13. Why should the hand be positioned higher than the elbow when a sling is applied?

    - promote circulation
    - prevent swelling
    - decrease pain

14. List four (4) points you can check to make sure that circulation is not impaired after a splint or sling has been applied.

    1) skin temperature   3) swelling

    2) skin color   4) amount of pain

15. What should you do if you notice signs of impaired circulation after applying a splint?

    Re-wrap the splint looser.

16. Why is it best to avoid moving any victim who has a neck or spinal injury?

    Permanent damage resulting in paralysis can occur.

Name _____ Date _____

Evaluated by _____

DIRECTIONS: Practice providing first aid for bone and joint injuries according to the criteria listed. When you are ready for your final check, give this sheet to your instructor.

Providing First Aid for Bone and Joint Injuries	Points Possible	Peer Check Yes	No	PROFICIENT Final Check* Yes	No	Points Earned**	Comments
1. Follows priorities of care:							
Checks the scene	2						
Checks consciousness and breathing	2						
Calls emergency medical services	2						
Cares for victim	2						
Controls bleeding	2						
2. Observes victim for signs of bone or joint injury	3						
3. Immobilizes any injured area or suspected fracture and/or dislocation	3						
4. Applies splints:							
Selects appropriate splint material	3						
Uses splints that will immobilize joint above and below injured area	3						
Positions splints correctly to avoid pressure on injury	3						
Pads splints especially at bony areas	3						
Ties splints in place	3						
Avoids any unnecessary movement during application	3						
5. Applies air/inflatable splints as follows:							
Obtains correct splint	3						
Supports injured area while positioning splint	3						
Inflates splint correctly	3						
Checks inflation by pressing on splint with thumb	3						
6. Applies sling with triangular bandage:							
Provides support for arm while applying	3						
Positions bandage with long edge on uninjured side	3						
Brings lower end up over injured arm and over shoulder on injured side	3						
Ties bandage ends with square knot avoiding bony area of neck and places padding between knot and skin	3						

14:9 (cont.)

Providing First Aid for Bone and Joint Injuries	Points Possible	Peer Check		Final Check*		Points Earned**	Comments
		Yes	No	Yes	No		
Secures area by elbow with pin or by tying in knot	3						
Checks to be sure fingers exposed and hand elevated 5 to 6 inches above elbow	3						
7. Checks for signs of impaired circulation by noting the following:							
Pale or bluish color	2						
Cold to touch	2						
Swelling/edema	2						
Pain or pressure from splint/sling	2						
Numbness or tingling	2						
Poor return of pink color after blanching nails	2						
8. Loosens splint/sling if impaired circulation noted	4						
9. Observes for signs of shock and treats as needed	4						
10. Applies cold applications to reduce swelling and pain	4						
11. Positions victim in a comfortable position but avoids unnecessary movement and avoids all movement if neck or spine injury suspected	4						
12. Reassures victim while providing first aid care	4						
13. Obtains medical help as soon as possible	4						
Totals	100						

* Final Check: Instructor or authorized person evaluates.
** Points Earned: Points possible times each "yes" check.

ASSIGNMENT SHEET

Grade _____ Name _____

INTRODUCTION: This assignment will help you review the specific care given to victims with injuries to the eye, ear, nose, brain, chest, abdomen, and genital organs.

INSTRUCTIONS: Read the information on Providing First Aid for Specific Injuries. In the space provided print the word(s) that best completes the statement or answers the question.

1. Injuries to the eye always involve the danger of *vision loss*. A top priority of first aid care is to obtain the assistance of *an eye specialist*, preferably a/an *medical help*.

2. Briefly describe two (2) techniques that can be used to remove a foreign object that is floating free in the eye.
   1) draw the upper lid down over the lower lid (stimulates tears)
   2) grasp the eyelashes and raise the upper eyelid

3. If an object is embedded in the eye, what first aid care should be given?
   Make no attempt to remove it.

4. List the steps of first aid treatment that should be followed when an object is protruding from the eye.
   - make no attempt to remove it
   - support it by loosely applying dressings

5. How should you care for tissue torn from the ear?
   Save the torn tissue in sterile water or saline and send it to the emergency room with the victim.

6. How should you position a victim with cerebrospinal fluid draining from the ear?
   Place the victim on their side and slightly elevate the head and allow the fluid to drain.

7. List six (6) signs and symptoms of injuries to the brain.
   1) fluid draining from ear/nose   *4) visual disturbances*
   2) loss of conciousness   *5) pupils unequal size*
   3) headache   *6) muscle paralysis*

8. List four (4) aspects of first aid care for victims with brain injuries.
   1) keep the victim lying flat + treat for shock
   2) watch for signs of respiratory distress
   3) don't stop the flow of fluid
   4) don't give the victim any fluids

9. List three (3) causes of an epistaxis or nosebleed.
   1) change in altitude
   2) strenuous activity
   3) high blood pressure

10. How should you position a victim with a nosebleed?
    – Sitting position
    – head leaning slightly forward

11. What type of dressing should be applied to a sucking chest wound? Why?
    – airtight dressing
    – to prevent air flow in and out
    – aluminum foil, or plastic wrap should be used

12. How should you position a victim with a sucking chest wound?
    – on the injured side
    – head slightly elevated

13. List four (4) signs and symptoms of abdominal injuries.
    1) abdominal pain or tenderness   3) open wounds
    2) protruding organs   4) nausea/vomitting

14. How should you position a victim with an abdominal injury?
    – flat on the back
    – pillow/blanket under the knees
    – elevated head + shoulders

15. How should you care for abdominal organs protruding from a wound?
    – dressings mositened w/ sterile water/saline
    – cover dressings with plastic wrap
    – then cover w/ foil or towel

16. List four (4) principles of first aid for injuries to genital organs.
    1) control severe bleeding w/ sterile dressing + applied pressure
    2) treat the victim for shock
    3) don't remove any penetrating or inserted object
    4) save any torn tissue

Name _____ Date _____

Evaluated by _____

DIRECTIONS: Practice providing first aid for specific injuries according to the criteria listed. When you are ready for your final check, give this sheet to your instructor.

PROFICIENT

Providing First Aid for Specific Injuries	Points Possible	Peer Check Yes	No	Final Check* Yes	No	Points Earned**	Comments
1. Follows priorities of care:							
Checks the scene	1						
Checks consciousness and breathing	1						
Calls emergency medical services	1						
Cares for victim	1						
Controls bleeding	1						
2. Observes victim for signs and symptoms of specific injuries	2						
3. Provides first aid for eye injuries:							
Washes hands thoroughly	2						
Removes free floating foreign object:							
Draws upper lid down over lower lid	2						
Raises upper lid and removes object with sterile gauze or gently flushes eye with water	2						
Applies sterile dressing if object embedded or above techniques do not work on free floating object	2						
If an object is protruding from the eye, immobilizes with dressings or cup with hole in bottom and makes no attempt to remove	2						
Covers both eyes with dressings to prevent movement of injured eye	2						
Positions victim lying flat	2						
Obtains medical help	2						
4. Provides first aid for ear injuries as follows:							
Applies light pressure with sterile dressing to control bleeding	2						
Preserves torn tissue by putting in sterile water or normal saline or gauze moistened with sterile water or normal saline	2						
Places sterile gauze loosely in outer ear canal for perforation of eardrum	2						
If cerebrospinal fluid is draining from ear:							
Avoids any attempt to stop flow	2						

Providing First Aid for Specific Injuries	Points Possible	Peer Check Yes	Peer Check No	Final Check* Yes	Final Check* No	Points Earned**	Comments
Positions victim on injured side with head and shoulders elevated slightly	2						
Positions dressing to absorb flow	2						
Obtains medical help	2						
5. Provides first aid for brain injuries as follows:							
Positions victim lying flat	2						
Elevates head and shoulders if no neck/spine injury	2						
Watches closely for respiratory distress	2						
Allows cerebrospinal fluid to drain and absorbs with dressings	2						
Avoids fluids—moistens lips, tongue and mouth with cool wet cloth if necessary	2						
Notes length of time the victim is unconscious	2						
Obtains medical help	2						
6. Provides first aid for nosebleed:							
Positions victim sitting with head leaning slightly forward	2						
Presses bleeding nostril(s) to midline	2						
If bleeding does not stop, inserts gauze in nostril(s) and applies pressure	2						
Applies cold wet compress or covered ice bag to bridge of nose	2						
Obtains medical help if bleeding does not stop, fracture suspected, or victim has repeated nosebleeds	2						
7. Provides first aid for chest injuries as follows:							
For sucking chest wound:							
Applies airtight dressing using aluminum foil or plastic and tapes on 3 sides	3						
Positions victim on injured side and elevates head and chest slightly	2						
For penetrating object:							
If object protruding, immobilizes in place and makes no attempt to remove it	3						
Positions victim in comfortable position but avoids unnecessary movement	2						
Watches closely for respiratory distress	2						
Obtains medical help immediately	2						

225

Providing First Aid for Specific Injuries	Points Possible	Peer Check Yes	Peer Check No	Final Check* Yes	Final Check* No	Points Earned**	Comments
8. Provides first aid for abdominal injuries:							
Positions victim lying flat with knees flexed slightly	2						
Elevates head and shoulders slightly to aid breathing	2						
If organs protruding, covers organs with sterile dressing moistened with sterile water or normal saline and plastic wrap or foil	3						
Avoids giving oral fluids	2						
Obtains medical help immediately	2						
9. Provides first aid for injuries to genital organs as follows:							
Controls bleeding with direct pressure	2						
Positions victim lying flat with legs separated	2						
Preserves any torn tissue by placing it in sterile cool water or normal saline or in gauze moistened with sterile cool water or normal saline	2						
Applies cold compresses or covered ice bag	2						
Obtains medical help	2						
10. Observes all victims for signs of shock and treats for shock immediately	2						
11. Reassures victim while providing care; encourages victim to relax as much as possible	2						
Totals	100						

* Final Check: Instructor or authorized person evaluates.
** Points Earned: Points possible times each "yes" check.

ASSIGNMENT SHEET

Grade _____   Name _____

INTRODUCTION: Sudden illness can occur in any individual, and you should know the major facts regarding first aid. This assignment will help you review these facts.

INSTRUCTIONS: Review the information on Providing First Aid for Sudden Illness. In the space provided, print the word(s) that best completes the statement or answers the question.

1. Identify three (3) sources of information you can use to help determine what illness a victim has.
   1) the victim
   2) medical alert bracelet/necklace
   3) medical information card

2. List four (4) signs and symptoms of a heart attack.
   1) shortness of breath   3) weakness
   2) blue lips/nail color   4) radiating pain in shoulders, arms, neck, + jaw

3. List three (3) first aid treatments for a heart attack victim.
   1) encouraging the victim to relax
   2) placing the victim in a comfortable position
   3) obtaining medical help

4. List six (6) signs and symptoms of a stroke.
   1) numbness   4) mental confusion
   2) paralysis   5) slurred speech
   3) pupils unequal size   6) nausea

5. List three (3) first aid treatments for a stroke.
   1) maintaining respirations
   2) laying victim on back w/ head elevated
   3) avoid fluids by mouth

6. If early symptoms of fainting are noted, how should you position the victim?
   - help victim to lie down or sit in a chair
   - place the head at the level of the knees

7. List three (3) points of first aid care for a victim who has fainted.
   1) elevate the victims legs 12 inches
   2) loosen any tight clothing
   3) maintain open airways

8. What is a convulsion?

A strong, involuntary contraction of muscles

9. First aid care for the victim with a convulsion is directed at preventing self-injury.

10. Should a padded tongue blade or soft object be placed between the victim's teeth during a convulsion? Why or why not?

-no
-can cause severe injury to your fingers
-can cause damage to the victims teeth/gums

11. Why is it important not to use force or restrain the muscle movements during a convulsion?

This can cause the contractions to become more severe.

12. In a victim with diabetes, an increase in the level of glucose or sugar in the blood can lead to a condition called diabetic coma, and an excess amount of insulin can lead to a condition called insulin shock.

13. List six (6) signs and symptoms of diabetic coma.

1) confusion
2) weakness
3) nausea
4) rapid, deep respirations
5) dry, flushed skin
6) sweet, fruity odor to breath

14. What is the main treatment for diabetic coma?

Call for medical assistance as quickly as possible.

15. List six (6) signs and symptoms of insulin shock.

1) muscle weakness
2) mental confusion
3) restlessness
4) diaphoresis
5) pale, moist skin
6) hungar pangs

16. What is the main treatment for insulin shock?

- a drink containing sugar

Name _____   Date _____

Evaluated by _____

DIRECTIONS: Practice providing first aid for sudden illness according to the criteria listed. When you are ready for your final check, give this sheet to your instructor.

PROFICIENT

Providing First Aid for Sudden Illness	Points Possible	Peer Check Yes	No	Final Check* Yes	No	Points Earned**	Comments
1. Follows priorities of care:							
Checks the scene	2						
Checks consciousness and breathing	2						
Calls emergency medical services	2						
Cares for victim	2						
Controls bleeding	2						
2. Observes victim for specific signs and symptoms of sudden illnesses	3						
3. Obtains information from victim regarding illness	3						
4. Checks for medical bracelet, necklace or card if victim unconscious	3						
5. Provides first aid for **heart attack** as follows:							
Positions in most comfortable position for victim	3						
Encourages relaxation	2						
Watches for signs of shock and treats as needed	2						
Moistens lips and mouth with wet cloth or gives small sips of water but avoids ice or cold water	2						
Obtains medical help as quickly as possible	2						
6. Provides first aid for **stroke** as follows:							
Positions in comfortable position	2						
Elevates head and shoulders to aid breathing	2						
Positions on side if victim having difficulty swallowing or unconscious	2						
Reassures victim and encourages relaxation	2						
Avoids fluids—moistens lips and mouth if necessary	2						
Obtains medical help immediately	2						

Providing First Aid for Sudden Illness	Points Possible	Peer Check Yes	No	Final Check* Yes	No	Points Earned**	Comments
7. Provides first aid for **fainting:**							
Keeps victim lying flat with feet raised if possible	3						
Loosens tight clothing	2						
Bathes face with cool water	2						
Checks for other injuries	2						
Encourages victim to lie flat until color improves	2						
After recovery, allows victim to get up slowly	3						
Obtains medical help if recovery delayed, other injuries noted, or other instances of fainting	2						
8. Provides first aid for **convulsions** as follows:							
Removes dangerous objects or moves victim if objects too heavy to move	3						
Places pillow, blanket, or soft object under head	3						
Checks respirations	2						
Avoids restraining muscle movements	2						
Notes length of convulsion and parts of body involved	2						
Watches closely after convulsion ends	2						
Obtains medical assistance if necessary	2						
9. Provides first aid for **diabetic coma** as follows:							
Positions in comfortable position or on side if unconscious	3						
Checks respirations closely	3						
Obtains medical help immediately	3						
10. Provides first aid for **insulin shock** as follows:							
Gives conscious victim drink with sugar	3						
Places sugar under tongue of unconscious victim	3						
Positions in comfortable position or on side if unconscious	3						
Obtains medical help if recovery not prompt	2						
11. Observes for signs of shock and treats as needed	3						
12. Reassures victim while providing care	3						
Totals	100						

* Final Check: Instructor or authorized person evaluates.
** Points Earned: Points possible times each "yes" check.

CHAPTER 14:12 APPLYING DRESSINGS AND BANDAGES

ASSIGNMENT SHEET

Grade _____   Name _____

INTRODUCTION: This assignment will help you review the main facts on dressings and bandages.

INSTRUCTIONS: Review the information on Applying Dressings and Bandages. In the space provided, print the word(s) that best completes the statement or answers the question.

1. What is a dressing?
   A sterile covering placed over a wound or injured part.

2. List three (3) purposes or functions of dressings.
   1) control bleeding
   2) absorb blood + secretions
   3) prevent infections

3. Why should you avoid using fluff cotton as a dressing?
   The loose cotton fibers may contaminate the wound.

4. What are bandages?
   Materials used to hold dressings in place, secure splints, and support and protect body parts.

5. Bandages should be applied snugly enough to control *bleeding* and prevent *movement of the dressing*, but not so tightly that they interfere with *circulation*.

6. List three (3) types or examples of bandages.
   1) roller gauze
   2) triangular
   3) elastic

7. List three (3) uses for triangular bandages.
   1) secure dressings on the head/scalp as slings
   2) covering for a large body part
   3) to secure splints/dressings

8. Why are elastic bandages hazardous?
   They can cut off or constrict circulation.

9. List four (4) signs that indicate poor circulation.
   1) swelling   *3) coldness*
   2) pale/blue shin   *4) numbness*

10. If any signs of impaired or poor circulation are noted after a bandage has been applied, what should you do?
    Immediately loosen the bandage.

Name _____ Date _____

Evaluated by _____

DIRECTIONS: Practice applying dressings and bandages according to the criteria listed. When you are ready for your final check, give this sheet to your instructor.

PROFICIENT

Applying Dressings and Bandages	Points Possible	Peer Check Yes	No	Final Check* Yes	No	Points Earned**	Comments
1. Assembles supplies	1						
2. Washes hands and puts on gloves	1						
3. Applies dressing as follows:							
Obtains correct size dressing	2						
Opens package without touching dressing	2						
Uses pinching action to pick up dressing	2						
Touches only one part of outside	2						
Holds dressing over wound and lowers onto wound	2						
Secures dressing with tape or bandage	2						
4. Applies triangular bandage to head or scalp:							
Folds two-inch hem in base	2						
Places sterile dressing on wound	2						
Positions middle of base on forehead with hem on outside	2						
Brings ends around head, above ears, crosses in back, and returns to forehead	2						
Ties ends in center of forehead with square knot	2						
Supports head while pulling point down in back to make bandage snug	2						
Tucks point into area where bandage crosses in back	2						
5. Folds a cravat with a triangular bandage:							
Brings point down to base	2						
Folds lengthwise until desired width obtained	2						
6. Applies circular bandage with cravat as follows:							
Places sterile dressing on wound	2						
Places center of cravat over dressing	2						
Carries ends around area and crosses when they meet	2						
Brings ends back to starting point	2						
Ties ends with square knot	2						

14:12 (cont.)

Applying Dressings and Bandages	Points Possible	Peer Check Yes	No	Final Check* Yes	No	Points Earned**	Comments
7. Applies spiral wrap with roller gauze:							
Places sterile dressing on wound	2						
Holds bandage with loose end coming off bottom	2						
Starts at bottom of limb and moves upward	2						
Anchors bandage correctly	2						
Circles area with spiral motion	2						
Overlaps each turn $\frac{1}{2}$ width of bandage	2						
Ends with 1 or 2 circular turns around limb	2						
Secures with tape, pins, or by tying	2						
8. Applies figure-eight wrap as follows:							
Places sterile dressing on wound	2						
Anchors bandage on instep	2						
Circles foot once or twice	2						
Angles over top of foot	2						
Goes behind ankle	2						
Circles down over top of foot and under instep	2						
Repeats pattern overlapping each turn $\frac{1}{2}$ to $\frac{2}{3}$ width of bandage	2						
Ends with 1 or 2 circular wraps around ankle	2						
Secures with tape, pins, or by tying	2						
9. Applies bandage to finger as follows:							
Places dressing on wound	2						
Holds gauze with loose end coming off bottom of roll	2						
Overlaps bandage on finger with 3–4 recurrent folds	2						
Uses spiral wrap to hold folds in position	2						
Uses figure-eight wrap around wrist to secure	2						
Ends by circling wrist	2						
Ties at wrist	2						
10. Checks circulation in area below bandage by noting following points:							
Pale or bluish	1						
Swelling	1						
Coldness	1						
Numbness or tingling	1						
Poor return of color after nail beds pressed lightly	1						
11. Loosens bandage immediately if any signs of impaired circulation noted	2						
12. Obtains medical help for victim as soon as possible	2						
13. Removes gloves and washes hands	1						
Totals	100						

* Final Check: Instructor or authorized person evaluates.
** Points Earned: Points possible times each "yes" check.

ASSIGNMENT SHEET

Grade _____ Name _____

INTRODUCTION: To keep a job, it will be essential for you to learn job-keeping skills. This assignment will help you evaluate your job-keeping skills.

INSTRUCTIONS: Read the information on Developing Job-Keeping Skills. In the space provided, print the word(s) that best completes the statement or answers the question.

1. Identify ten (10) deficiencies that employers feel are common in high school students.

2. Choose at least three (3) job-keeping skills for which you feel you are proficient. Give at least two (2) reasons why you feel you are competent in each of the skills.

3. Choose at least three (3) job-keeping skills for which you feel you need improvement. Explain why you are not competent in these skills. Then identify at least two (2) ways you can improve your competency in each of these skills.

ASSIGNMENT SHEET

Grade _____ Name _____

INTRODUCTION: A letter of application and a resumé are two important parts of obtaining employment. This assignment will help you review the main facts regarding the letter and resumé.

INSTRUCTIONS: Read the information on Writing a Letter of Application and Resumé. In the space provided print the word(s) that best completes the statement or answers the question.

1. What is the main purpose of the letter of application?

2. The letter should be _____ on good quality paper. It must be
_____, _____, and done according to correct _____
for letters. Care must be taken to ensure that _____ and _____ are
correct.

3. Briefly state the contents for each of the paragraphs in a letter of application.

   a. paragraph 1:

   b. paragraph 2:

   c. paragraph 3:

   d. paragraph 4:

4. What is a resumé?

5. Briefly list the type of information found in each of the following parts of a resumé.

   a. personal identification:

   b. employment objective:

   c. educational background:

   d. work or employment experience:

   e. skills:

   f. other activities:

   g. references:

6. Why is honesty always the best policy when completing resumés?

7. What type of envelope should you use to mail the letter of application and resumé?

8. What is the purpose of a career passport or portfolio?

   List five (5) items that might be included in a career passport or portfolio.

9. List the three (3) foundation skills recognized by SCANS.

10. Choose three (3) of the SCANS workplace competencies. For each competency, write a brief explanation of how you have mastered it.

CHAPTER 15:2 INVENTORY SHEET FOR RESUMÉS

Grade _____ Name _____

INTRODUCTION: The following information is required for resumés.

INSTRUCTIONS: Use a telephone book, address books, school records, and other sources to complete the following information about yourself.

Name _____

Address _____
            Number & Street   City   State   Zip

Telephone ( ) _____ Social Security _____

Name of School _____

School Address _____
            No. & Street   City   State   Zip

Dates of Attendance _____

Degree Earned _____ Major _____

Special Skills Learned _____

Computer Skills/Courses _____

Grade Average _____ Awards Earned _____

_____

_____

Other Schools Attended: Name _____

    Address _____

Previous Employers: Most recent first

Names	Address City, State, Zip	Dates of Employment	Duties Job Titles

References: Names (at least 3)   Full Address and Telephone   Title

_____

_____

_____

Other Activities: Include clubs, offices, volunteer work, hobbies

_____

_____

_____

Name _____ Date _____

Evaluated by _____

DIRECTIONS: Practice writing a letter of application according to the criteria listed. When you are ready for your final check, give this sheet to your instructor along with the letter of application.

PROFICIENT

Writing a Letter of Application	Points Possible	Peer Check Yes	No	Final Check* Yes	No	Points Earned**	Comments
1. Uses good quality paper	6						
2. Computer prints or types all information neatly and accurately	6						
3. Follows correct form for either block or modified block style letters	6						
4. Completes contents of letter as follows:							
Addresses to correct individual	8						
States purpose for writing	8						
States position applying for	8						
Lists source of advertisement or referring person	8						
States why qualified	8						
States resumé enclosed or furnished on request	8						
Includes information on how employer can contact	8						
Asks for interview and thanks employer for considering application	8						
5. Spells all words correctly	6						
6. Punctuates all information and sentences correctly	6						
7. Uses complete sentences and correct grammar	6						
Totals	100						

* Final Check: Instructor or authorized person evaluates.
** Points Earned: Points possible times each "yes" check.

Name _____   Date _____

Evaluated by _____

DIRECTIONS: Practice writing a resumé according to the criteria listed. When you are ready for your final check, give this sheet to your instructor along with the resumé.

Writing a Resumé	Points Possible	Peer Check Yes	No	Final Check* Yes	No	Points Earned**	Comments
1. Uses good quality paper	6						
2. Computer prints or types all information neatly and accurately	6						
3. Follows consistent format and spacing throughout resumé	6						
4. Includes all the following information:							
Personal identification: name, address, telephone	10						
Employment objective	10						
Educational background: name and address of school, special courses, or training	10						
Work or employment experience: name and address of employers, dates employed, job title, description of duties, in order from most recent backward	10						
Skills and specific knowledge	10						
Other activities: organizations, offices held, awards, volunteer work, hobbies, interests	10						
References: full name, title, and address or states "References will be furnished on request"	10						
5. Spells all words correctly	6						
6. Punctuates all information correctly	6						
Totals	100						

* Final Check: Instructor or authorized person evaluates.
** Points Earned: Points possible times each "yes" check.

CHAPTER 15:3 COMPLETING JOB APPLICATION FORMS

ASSIGNMENT SHEET #1

Grade _____ Name _____

INTRODUCTION: This assignment will help you review the main facts about completing job application forms.

INSTRUCTIONS: Read the information about Completing Job Application Forms. In the space provided, print the word(s) that best completes the statement or answers the question.

1. Why do employers use job application forms?

2. List three (3) reasons why you should read the application form completely before you fill in the information.

3. If questions do not apply to you, what should you put in the space provided for the answer to the question?

4. Why is it important to watch spelling and punctuation?

5. If the application does not state otherwise, it is best to type or _____. Use _____ if printing.

6. Why must all information be correct and truthful?

7. If a space is labeled "office use only," how do you complete this section? Why?

8. What should you do before using anyone's name as a reference?

9. What is the purpose of the wallet card?

10. Identify three (3) things you should look for when you proofread your completed application.

CHAPTER 15:3 COMPLETING JOB APPLICATION FORMS: WALLET CARD

ASSIGNMENT SHEET # 2

Grade _____ Name _____

INTRODUCTION: When you are looking for a job, you must be prepared. To be sure that you always have the needed information, it is wise to carry a "wallet card" with you. A sample form is given.

INSTRUCTIONS: Complete the information listed. This is information that can be used during job interviews but most of the time it is required for application forms. The sheet can be glued to an index card and kept in your wallet for easy reference. The information may also be written on a small index card.

Registration/License number _____ Social Security _____

Grade School Name _____

      Address _____ Zip _____

      Date Attended _____

Junior High Name _____

      Address _____ Zip _____

      Date Attended _____

High School Name _____

      Address _____ Zip _____

      Date Attended _____

Special Training—Major _____

Computer Skills/ Courses _____

Activities _____

Special Skills _____

_____

Employment:

Dates	Name	Position	Full Address and Telephone	Salary

References: Include name, title, full address, telephone (Include at least 3)

_____

_____

_____

Other Facts _____

_____

ASSIGNMENT SHEET #3

Grade _____ Name _____

INTRODUCTION: To obtain a job, you will probably have to complete an application form. The sample form that follows will help prepare you for this task.

INSTRUCTIONS: Review the information about Completing Job Application Forms. Complete the information on your "wallet card." Then use this information to complete the following form.

Health Careers Unlimited Application

Please type or print all information required. Be sure all information is accurate and complete.

Name in Full _____

Full Address _____

City _____ State _____ Zip _____

Social Security _____ Telephone _____

Position Desired _____

What prompted you to apply here? _____

When will you be available to start work? _____

Will you work (check if yes) any shift? _____ Holidays? _____

      Weekends? _____ Part-time? _____ Full Time? _____

Salary Expected _____ Registration Number _____

Education: (Circle last grade completed)

High School   1   2   3   4   Name _____

      From _____ Address in Full _____

      To _____ _____

College   1   2   3   4   Name _____

      From _____ Address in Full _____

      To _____ _____

Military Record: Branch of Service _____

      Date Entered _____ Date Discharged _____

      Discharge Status _____ Rank _____

Activities/Organizations/Special Skills _____

Computer Skills/Courses _____

Employment Record (list most recent position first)

Name of Employer _____

Full Address _____

Telephone _____ Dates: From _____ To _____

Supervisor's Name _____

Average Salary _____ Job Title _____

Reason for Leaving _____

Name of Employer _____

Full Address _____

Telephone _____ Dates: From _____ To _____

Supervisor's Name _____

Average Salary _____ Job Title _____

Reason for Leaving _____

Name of Employer _____

Full Address _____

Telephone _____ Dates: From _____ To _____

Supervisor's Name _____

Average Salary _____ Job Title _____

Reason for Leaving _____

References: List names, titles, full address, and telephone

1. _____

   _____

2. _____

   _____

3. _____

   _____

I affirm that all of these statements are true and correct. I grant permission for verification of any of these fact

Date _____ Signature _____

Do not write below this line:

Date Interviewed _____ Position _____

Salary _____ Starting Date _____ Initials _____

Name _____ Date _____

Evaluated by _____

DIRECTIONS: Practice completing job application forms according to the criteria listed. When you are ready for your final check, give this sheet to your instructor.

PROFICIENT

Completing Job Application Forms	Points Possible	Peer Check Yes	No	Final Check* Yes	No	Points Earned**	Comments
1. Completes wallet card correctly:							
Prints or types neatly	8						
Inserts accurate information	8						
Lists full addresses, zip codes, names, etc.	8						
2. Types or prints in black ink on application form unless writing requested on form	7						
3. Follows all directions provided on form completely	8						
4. Completes all of the following information on form:							
Personal information	8						
Education	8						
Work experience	8						
References	8						
Signature in correct area	8						
5. Spells all words correctly	7						
6. Leaves "office space" and similar areas blank	7						
7. Completes form neatly and thoroughly; places "none" or "NA" in spaces as necessary	7						
Totals	100						

* Final Check: Instructor or authorized person evaluates.
** Points Earned: Points possible times each "yes" check.

CHAPTER 15:4 PARTICIPATING IN A JOB INTERVIEW

ASSIGNMENT SHEET

Grade _____   Name _____

INTRODUCTION: A job interview is an essential part of obtaining a job. This assignment will review the main facts.

INSTRUCTIONS: Review the information on Participating in a Job Interview. In the space provided, print the word(s) that best completes the statement or answers the question.

1. List two (2) purposes of the job interview.

2. List two (2) things containing information that you should take to the job interview with you.

3. List four (4) rules for dress or appearance that should be observed.

4. How early should you arrive for a job interview?

5. List eight (8) rules of conduct that should be observed during a job interview.

6. What should you do after the job interview to let the employer know you are still interested in the position?

7. Write a brief response to each of the following questions as though you were being asked during a job interview.

   a. "Why do you feel you are qualified for this position?"

   b. "What are your strengths or strong points?"

   c. "I see you recently got married. Do you plan to start a family soon?"

   d. "What do you feel are the three most important features of a job?"

   e. "What do you hope to accomplish during the next two years?"

Name _____ Date _____

Evaluated by _____

DIRECTIONS: Practice participating in a job interview according to the criteria listed. When you are ready for your final check, give this sheet to your instructor.

PROFICIENT

Participating in a Job Interview	Points Possible	Peer Check Yes	No	Final Check* Yes	No	Points Earned**	Comments
1. Dresses appropriately for interview	6						
2. Prepares wallet card, resumé, job application	5						
3. Arrives 5–10 minutes early for interview	5						
4. Introduces self to employer and shakes hands firmly if indicated	5						
5. Refers to employer by name	5						
6. Sits correctly with good posture	5						
7. Listens closely to employer's questions and comments	6						
8. Answers all questions thoroughly but keeps answers pertinent	6						
9. Speaks slowly and clearly without mumbling	6						
10. Smiles when appropriate but avoids excessive laughter or giggling	5						
11. Maintains eye contact with employer	6						
12. Avoids mannerisms during interview	6						
13. Uses correct English and avoids slang terms	6						
14. Uses correct manners and acts polite	6						
15. Avoids smoking, chewing gum, eating candy, and so forth	5						
16. Asks questions pertaining to job responsibility and avoids questioning fringe benefits, raises, and so forth	6						
17. Thanks employer for the interview at the end	6						
18. Shakes hands firmly if indicated	5						
Totals	100						

* Final Check: Instructor or authorized person evaluates.

** Points Earned: Points possible times each "yes" check.

ASSIGNMENT SHEET

Grade _____ Name _____

INTRODUCTION: To determine how much money you have available after deductions, you must figure out your net income. This assignment will help you do this.

INSTRUCTIONS: Follow the instructions in each of the following sections. Place your answers in the blanks on the right. Double-check all figures for accuracy. Your instructor will supply an hourly wage rate if you are not employed.

1. List your wage per hour (how much you make an hour).

   1. _____

2. Multiply your wage per hour times the number of hours you work per week. Usually a 40 hour work week is an average amount.

   Wage Per Hour × Hours Worked Per Week =

   2. _____

   This amount is your gross weekly pay.

3. Determine the average deductions that will be taken out of your gross weekly pay.

   a. Determine deduction for federal tax by multiplying the gross pay times the percentage of deduction found on federal tax tables. (An average amount is 15 percent or 0.15.)

      _____ × _____ =
      Gross Pay   Federal Tax Percentage

      a. _____

   b. Determine deduction for state tax by multiplying the gross pay times the percentage of deduction found on state tax tables. (An average amount is 2 percent or 0.02.)

      _____ × _____ =
      Gross Pay   State Tax Percentage

      b. _____

   c. Determine deduction for city/corporation tax by multiplying the gross pay times the percentage found on city tax tables. (An average amount is 1 percent or 0.01.)

      _____ × _____ =
      Gross Pay   City Tax Percentage

      c. _____

   d. Determine the deduction for FICA or Social Security by multiplying gross pay times the current deduction. (Use 7.65 percent or 0.0765 if unknown.)

      _____ × _____ =
      Gross Pay   Social Security Percentage

      d. _____

e. List any other deductions that are subtracted from your gross pay. This can include payments for insurance, charity, union dues, and so forth. Add all these deductions together to get the total for miscellaneous deductions.

e. _____

_____

_____

f. Add the answers in a., b., c., d., and e. together to get the total amount of deductions.

f. _____

4. Subtract the amount in answer 3.f. (total amount of all deductions) from the gross weekly pay listed in question 2. This amount will be your net weekly pay or "take home" weekly pay.

_____ – _____ = _____   4. _____

  Gross Pay   Deductions   Net Weekly Pay

5. To determine your net pay per month, multiply the weekly net pay times 4 for four week months. Multiply the weekly net pay times 5 for five week months.

_____ × _____ = _____   5. _____

  Net Weekly Pay   Weeks Per Month   Net Monthly Pay

Note: The weekly net pay can be multiplied by 52 weeks to determine yearly net pay.

Name _____ Date _____

Evaluated by _____

DIRECTIONS: Practice determining net income according to the criteria listed. When you are ready for your final check, give this sheet to your instructor.

PROFICIENT

Determining Net Income	Points Possible	Peer Check Yes	No	Final Check* Yes	No	Points Earned**	Comments
1. Lists wage per hour	10						
2. Determines gross weekly pay by multiplying wage per hour times the number of hours worked per week	14						
3. Determines deduction for federal tax by multiplying correct percentage times gross weekly pay	10						
4. Determines deduction for state tax by multiplying correct percentage times gross weekly pay	10						
5. Determines deduction for city/corporation tax by multiplying correct percentage times gross weekly pay	10						
6. Determines deduction for social security by multiplying correct percentage times gross weekly pay	10						
7. Lists any miscellaneous deductions and obtains a total for these by adding all miscellaneous deductions together	10						
8. Adds amounts for federal tax, state tax, city/corporation tax, social security, and miscellaneous deductions together	12						
9. Subtracts total amount of deductions from gross weekly pay to get net weekly pay	14						
Totals	100						

* Final Check: Instructor or authorized person evaluates.
** Points Earned: Points possible times each "yes" check.

CHAPTER 15:6 CALCULATING A BUDGET

ASSIGNMENT SHEET

Grade _____ Name _____

INTRODUCTION: To avoid financial problems, planning and foresight is required. This assignment will help you prepare a budget and plan monthly expenses. Follow the instructions in each section to calculate a budget.

1. List monthly expenses for the following items:

   Rent (you may have to share an apartment)   _____

   Utilities: heat, electricity, telephone, water, garbage, and so forth   _____

   Food:include all food items purchased, money for food away from home   _____

   Car Expenses:

       Gasoline   _____

       Insurance (divide yearly payment by 12)   _____

       Oil, maintenance, tires, repairs   _____

       Payment for purchase   _____

       Other: (note what)   _____

   Laundry or cleaning of clothes   _____

   Clothing purchase (include uniforms)   _____

   Payments: Furniture   _____

             Charge accounts   _____

             Other bills   _____

   Personal items: shampoo, toothpaste, and so forth   _____

   Donations: Church, charities   _____

   Medical or Life Insurance payments (divide yearly payment by 12)   _____

   Education expenses (fees, books, and so forth)   _____

   Savings (strive for 10%)   _____

   Other items: List   _____   _____

                   _____   _____

   Entertainment, hobbies, and so forth   _____

   Miscellaneous: "Mad" money, and so forth   _____

                                                                TOTAL 1. $ _____

2. List your net pay per four week month.

                                                                TOTAL 2. $ _____

3. If the total in number 2 is larger than the total in number 1, you may add more money to items in your budget. If number 1 is larger, you have overspent. Refigure your budget. Figure in number 1 should equal figure in number 2 for a balanced budget.

Name _____ Date _____

Evaluated by _____

DIRECTIONS: Practice calculating a budget according to the criteria listed. When you are ready for your final check, give this sheet to your instructor.

PROFICIENT

Calculating a Budget	Points Possible	Peer Check Yes	No	Final Check* Yes	No	Points Earned**	Comments
1. Lists realistic monthly amounts for each of the following items:							
Rent or house payments	5						
Utilities	5						
Food	5						
Car expenses:							
Gasoline	3						
Insurance (divides yearly payment by 12)	3						
Oil, maintenance, and so forth	3						
Payment for purchase	3						
Laundry or cleaning of clothes	5						
Clothing purchase	5						
Payments:							
Furniture	3						
Charge accounts	3						
Other bills	3						
Personal items	5						
Donations	5						
Medical or life insurance (divides yearly payment by 12)	5						
Education expenses	5						
Savings	5						
Entertainment, hobbies	5						
Miscellaneous expenses	5						
2. Determines net monthly income accurately	6						
3. Totals all expenses in budget for total monthly expenses accurately	6						
4. Balances budget by making monthly expenses equal net monthly income	7						
Totals	100						

* Final Check: Instructor or authorized person evaluates.
** Points Earned: Points possible times each "yes" check.

CHAPTER 16 COMPUTERS IN HEALTH CARE

ASSIGNMENT SHEET

Grade _____ Name _____

INTRODUCTION: The computer has become an essential ingredient in almost every aspect of health care. This assignment will help you review the main facts about computers.

INSTRUCTIONS: Read the information on Computers in Health Care. In the space provided, print the word(s) that best completes the statement or answers the question.

1. Name four (4) general areas of health care that use computers.

2. Define *computer literacy*.

3. List at least eight (8) commonly used items that contain computer chips.

4. A computer system is a/an _____ device that can be thought of as a complete _____. It can _____, _____, _____, _____, _____, _____, _____, and _____ data.

5. What is the difference between hardware and software in computer systems?

6. Identify at least six (6) input devices that can be used to enter data into the computer.

7. What is the function of the central processing unit (CPU) of the computer?

8. What is the difference between the read only memory (ROM) and the random access memory (RAM) in the internal memory unit of a computer?

9. What is output?

   Name two (2) output devices.

10. Health care providers use computers to perform many functions. Identify at least five (5) of these functions.

11. How can confidentiality be maintained while using a computer for patient records?

12. What advantage does computerized tomography have over regular X-rays?

13. How does ultrasonography create an image of the body part such as a developing fetus?

14. What is the Internet?

    What is a major use for the Internet in health care?

15. The use of computers has introduced many new abbreviations. Identify the following abbreviations as they relate to computers.

    a. CAI

    b. CPU

    c. CRT

    d. CT

    e. HIS

    f. MIS

    g. MRI

    h. PET

    i. RAM

    j. ROM

CHAPTER 17 MEDICAL MATH

ASSIGNMENT SHEET

Grade _____ Name _____

INTRODUCTION: This assignment will help you review math concerns and concepts that are essential to working in health care.

INSTRUCTIONS: Read the information on Medical Math. In the space provided, print the word(s) that best completes the statement or answers the question.

1. Identify three (3) methods that can be used to overcome math anxiety?

2. _____ are what we traditionally use to count, they do not contain fractions or decimals. _____ are one way of expressing parts of numbers and are expressed in units of ten. _____ have a numerator and a denominator. It is easier to calculate _____ if you first convert them to decimals. _____ show relationships between numbers or like values: how many of one number of value is present as compared to the other. _____ a number means changing it to the nearest ten, hundred, thousand, and so on.

3. List four (4) guidelines to make estimating useful.

4. Perform the calculations indicated for whole numbers.

   a. $742 + 1,259 =$

   b. $1,138 + 1,423 + 2,557 + 924 =$

   c. $238,031 - 152,987 =$

   d. $18,654 - 8,986 =$

   e. $22 \times 156 =$

   f. $1,057 \times 324 =$

   g. $555 \div 15 =$

   h. $171,450 \div 9,525 =$

5. Perform the calculations indicated for decimals.

    a. $5.893 + 87.32 + 0.5 =$

    b. $54.5 + 0.05455 + 5450 + 5.00456 =$

    c. $78.3 - 49.538 =$

    d. $485.782 - 396.99 =$

    e. $28.561 \times 5.39 =$

    f. $0.614 \times 0.00568 =$

    g. $125.49 \div 2.35 =$

    h. $1027.08 \div 6.34 =$

6. Perform the calculations indicated for fractions.

    a. $1/8 + 3/4 + 1/2 =$

    b. $3\ 5/8 + 20\ 3/5 =$

    c. $15/16 - 3/8 =$

    d. $46\ 3/4 - 37\ 1/3 =$

    e. $7/12 \times 8/21 =$

    f. $12\ 2/5 \times 5\ 5/8 =$

    g. $7/8 \div 5/6 =$

    h. $27\ 1/2 \div 5\ 1/2 =$

7. Perform the calculations indicated for percentages.

    a. $38\% + 53.5\% =$

    b. $54.3\% - 11.4\% =$

    c. $230 \times 5\% =$

    d. $563 \div 2\% =$

8. Round the following numbers to the place indicated.

    a. 9,837 to the nearest tenth =

    b. 652 to the nearest hundredth =

    c. 1,479 to the nearest thousandth =

9. Use proportions to calculate the following problems.

    a. How many 250 mg tablets must be given for a total dosage of 750 mg?

    b. How many 5 grain aspirins must be given for a total dosage of 7.5 grains?

    c. How many milligrams of medication should you give an 80 pound person if dosage requires 20 mg for every 10 pounds of weight?

    d. If 45 milliliters of water is required to mix 100 grams of plaster, how many milliliters would you need for 250 grams of plaster?

10. Convert the following numbers to Roman numerals.

    a. 55

    b. 109

    c. 595

    d. 788

    e. 2367

11. Interpret the following Roman numerals.

    a. XII

    b. CCXIX

    c. XLIV

    d. DCXCII

    e. MMMDXXXIII

12. Give three (3) examples of how angles are used in health care.

13. What are the six (6) steps used for performing conversions between systems of measurement?

14. Convert the following as indicated. Use the approximate equivalents shown in the textbook to calculate your answers.

    a. 5 teaspoons = ? milliliters

    b. 1250 milliliters = ? quarts

    c. 33 kilograms = ? pounds

    d. 6 ounces = ? milliliters

    e. 121 pounds = ? kilograms

    f. 2 feet = ? centimeters

15. Convert the following temperatures from Fahrenheit to Celsius and round off the answer to the nearest one-tenth of a degree.

    a. 35°F

    b. 72°F

    c. 99.6°F

    d. 103°F

16. Convert the following temperatures from Celsius to Fahrenheit and round off the answer to the nearest one-tenth of a degree.

    a. 30°C

    b. 62°C

    c. 15°C

    d. 25.6°C

17. Define *military time.*

18. Convert the following to military time.

    a. 1:00 PM

    b. 2:00 AM

    c. 12:00 NOON

    d. 3:00 AM

    e. 8:35 PM

    f. 5:05 AM

    g. 11:48 PM

    h. 12:00 MIDNIGHT

INDEX